YOGA
GIRLS' CLUB

YOGA
GIRLS' CLUB

Do Yoga, Make Art, Be You

TIFFANI BRYANT

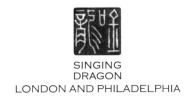

SINGING
DRAGON
LONDON AND PHILADELPHIA

First published in 2015
by Singing Dragon
an imprint of Jessica Kingsley Publishers
73 Collier Street
London N1 9BE, UK
and
400 Market Street, Suite 400
Philadelphia, PA 19106, USA

www.singingdragon.com

Library of Congress Cataloging in Publication Data
A CIP catalog record for this book is available from the Library of Congress

British Library Cataloguing in Publication Data
A CIP catalogue record for this book is available from the British Library

ISBN 978 1 84819 259 1
eISBN 978 0 85701 206 7

Printed and bound in Great Britain

Turn your face to the sun and the shadows fall behind you.
MAORI PROVERB

We are more than the walls these forms perceive…
VYLINDA ANN BRYANT

ACKNOWLEDGMENTS

Thank you, Lord, for filling me with your light and showing me that all is possible with faith, patience, and believing. Vylinda Ann Bryant, I could not exist without your love, inspiration, and creative dreaming; thank you for being my best friend through it all. Singing Dragon and Jessica Kingsley Publishers, thank you for giving this work wings.

CONTENTS

INTRODUCTION

Welcome to *Yoga Girls' Club*, an ever-expanding community for us. *Yoga Girls' Club* is a guide, canvas, and suitcase where you can begin to collect, reflect on, and express the pieces that form you. Once, when my vacation was ending and I was walking toward the connecting tram to the airport, a girl with an afro as big as the sun and eyes as near and far away as the sky was walking toward me pulling a large suitcase. She said, "We're all on a journey." She was right.

Being a part of this club is fun and work. The requirements: a commitment to finding your best flow (the way you move through the world), taking responsibility for finding and being the best you—making this a regular (daily, hourly, step-by-step) practice and maintaining a spirit of adventure. You are a beautiful work of art, part physical, part spiritual, part emotion, part mystery; you have infinite possibilities.

This journey begins with getting to know who you are, inside and out, as you move through the places, spaces, and roles of your life. There is no one else exactly like you, so it is your responsibility to *discover* and *be* your best self. What lights you up and makes you happy? What areas do you need to grow as you tend the garden of *you*? How do you flow through your world? Shining and positive or like a cloudy day and negative? What feels most like *you*? Do you know what makes you spiral out of control toward great highs or low lows? What would happen if you were in charge of how this feels inside, and eventually how it looks (to you and others) on the outside?

On these pages you will practice yoga and learn more about yourself. You will explore your creative side—it might be subtle, it might be bold; it's there, it's part of you.

Yoga is full of metaphors. Look out for them in *Yoga Girls' Club*; they will help you feel the postures in your body, and see the possibilities in your mind.

Yoga Girls' Club Mantra

I will show up for myself.

I will keep an open mind as I learn more about myself.

I will treat myself with kindness.

I will shine my light, when it is as strong as the sun or as weak as one lightning bug.

I am happy to be me.

I am a Yoga Girl with an important mission in this world.

CHAPTER 1

Creating My Space

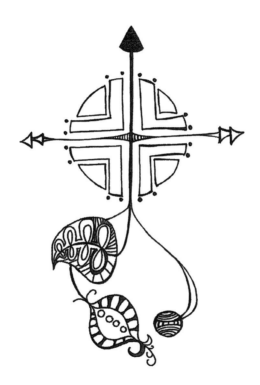

When you change yourself, you change the world.
Each journey begins with a step; what does your compass look like?

Within and outside *Yoga Girls' Club*, begin to create a space that is all your own. A space where you can relax and get away from the rest of the world (the chatter of other voices, the call of technology, the expectations of others), release any worries and concerns, and get comfortable with *you*.

You might already have your own special space carved out or you might need to begin searching for it. Wherever your space might be, let it be someplace that is not dependent on others or their ideas of what it should be; just feel (when you are in this place) it is your own.

Play some music or explore silence; more importantly, hear the rhythm of your own breath.

In this space, believe in yourself and your gifts. Know that only you can be you and that you are amazing.

Your space does not have to be a room that is your own. It can be a small piece of earth outside your back door, at the beach or a park where you can feel the sun on your skin, or a little bit of floor space next to a window. This space is in your head and heart, whether it exists physically outside of you or not.

No one has to know where your space is or how you get there, but when you enter your space, acknowledge: *I am filled with light, knowledge, and gifts to share.*

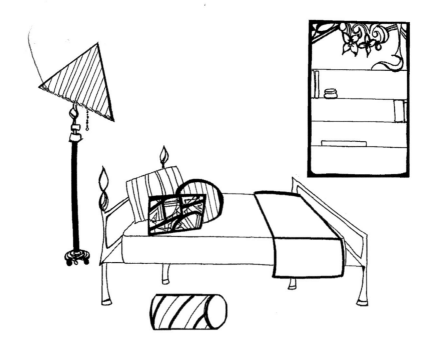

Wherever your space is, return to it over and over so
you can step right back into the energy you are building
on this journey. You may end up having many spaces,
since this energy travels in your head and heart.

Gathering Supplies

All you need for this journey within is an open mind and a spirit of adventure. Simply try. Observe what you experience and take it step by step without judgment or thinking that you cannot do something. If you try, you will find a world of things you can do.

For your yoga practice, you might need: a yoga mat, two yoga blocks, a yoga strap, and a blanket. You can always improvise, though. Be creative; use things you already have, give yourself enough floor space to move, and create a surface where you will not slip. A scarf with colors you like could be your yoga strap and a sweatshirt could be folded and rolled into a tight bundle to make your seat more comfortable or placed under your neck for support when you are lying down. A wall is also a friend when it comes to balancing postures.

For the creative projects, collect sources of color—markers, pens, and glitter. Make one of your intentions to write, draw, and personalize the pages of this book. Collect images from magazines, inspiration from television, movies, and the people around you. Avoid if possible easy comparisons that you can see. Try to start looking beneath and beyond the glittering surface of people, places, and things.

We're going to try to discover what these objects, images, concepts, and examples mean to you.

Under Construction

I am: A strong, powerful, motivated girl who knows who she wants to be and how she is going to get there.

My worldview is: Everybody desevers a fair chance and everyone deserves to be helped, because everyone is equal and equally as important.

You will reconstruct this page often.

Strive to stretch yourself, to become more you

How can I view and interact with the world differently?

_____

_____

_____

_____

How can I incorporate my practice of yoga into my thoughts, words, and actions?

_____

_____

_____

_____

How can I change my state of mind, when I feel as if my head is exploding?

_____

_____

_____

_____

How can I generate energy when I feel too sad, mad, or depressed to face my day?

_____

_____

_____

_____

How can I influence the world by shining the light of the young woman I know myself to be?

_____

_____

_____

_____

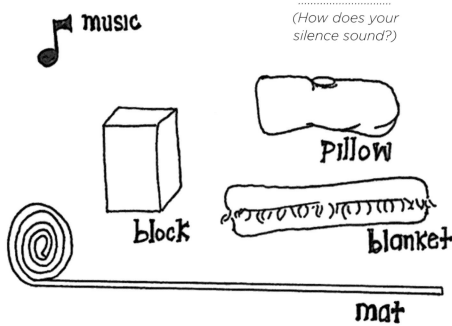

music

"............................."
(How does your silence sound?)

Pillow

block

blanket

mat

Your Yoga Tools

Coloring My World

Have you ever thought about the meaning of different colors? Ever notice how certain shades make you feel? Why do you gravitate toward a bright orange, yet dull green repels you? What does it all mean?

Green, blue, and violet are cool colors, while red, orange, and yellow are warm colors.

Over time and across cultures colors can express themselves in different ways depending on what people believe about particular shades and how they've seen them work in their lives and land. Color magic probably has a very similar place in your life. Color preference is personal. Do you notice how it lives and travels with you? In North America red is often associated with love, passion, and danger; black with negativity and sometimes sleekness, like a running panther; yellow with positivity; green with nature and growth, commerce, and wanting what someone else has; gray with the unknown; and white with clean, untouched space.

In your yoga practice, begin to think of the ways different colors are connected to your highs and lows: happy, angry, sad, tired, lonely, full, empty, heavy, weightless, unnoticed, important. How do your color choices affect and reflect you? As you make your art and express your personal style, the colors you use can help you say what you are trying to communicate.

Did you know that certain colors also form the rainbow of your energy? Your body has seven centers of energy called *chakras*. Beginning at the base of your spine running up to the crown of your head. Each *chakra* can spin fast with free-flowing energy or slow down and become sluggish because it's clogged with stuff you don't need. Is your energy standing still like a stopped up drain?

Colour Moods

Using a magazine that is ready to be discarded, cut out strong examples of red, orange, yellow, green, turquoise, indigo, and violet. Choose shades that say something to you.

| Glue color here | Red | *Root Chakra* Base of spine | Red can ground you and help you feel balanced and supported wherever you are. To begin to feel this support (like the ground beneath you) settle into your *Comfortable Seat*. Concentrate on your red square. Think about your home and the places you go. Do you have food to eat? Do you feel safe? Does your family love you? Do you love them? Do you have friends that make you laugh? Your red can be a source of power anytime you need to feel strong. |
| Glue color here | Orange | *Receptivity Chakra* Hips | Orange can inspire you to find your best flow, to get in touch with your feelings, to draw, write, dance, sing... whatever you do to express yourself creatively. This might sound funny, but sometimes it can feel like life is happening to us, determining whether we are victims or victors. If you remain open, aware, and strong as you notice what is going on, this *chakra* can help you experience your "best days" and have some control over how you move through good and bad times. |

Glue color here	Yellow	*Power Chakra* Pit of belly	Yellow can help you harness the power in your third *chakra*, the low part of your belly, where your sense of self lies. Close your eyes, look and feel beneath your outer layers of skin, then move through your muscles and bones to study yourself. Ask these questions: Am I more aware of "me?" Who am I? Who do I want to become? What do I want to do in the world? Asking yourself these questions can help you find your place at different points in your day, and life.
Glue color here	Green	*Connection Chakra* Heart	Green can open a space inside you, where you might be able to let go of things you've been holding, negative stuff that's blocking you. The heart *chakra* can help you define what "love" means to you, and how it is working in your relationships with others.
Glue color here	Turquoise	*Expression Chakra* Throat	Turquoise can help you decide what you really believe about many things: the people you interact with, what spirituality and religion mean to you, what you think about what's going on in the world. This process begins by making a definition for the word "truth." Dig deep; it's personal—it's inside you. Then, see how your truth works when a situation outside you asks you to act on what you really believe. Be flexible here, as you learn more about your place in the world, your truth can take new shapes like a yoga posture you hold for a while.

Glue color here	Indigo	*Intuition Chakra* Center of forehead	Indigo expands your ability to feel and know and understand from the inside: the pit of your belly, your heart, your throat. Think of it as an incredible eye in the center of your forehead. You can see, feel, and understand with its clear lens because it can see with your "truth" even when your eyes cannot.
Glue color here	Violet	*Higher Self Chakra* Crown of head	Violet clears your head and heart, creating room for you to feel like you can find your place. Wherever you go, the right shade of violet and the energy at the crown of your head can make you feel light, prepared, free from anything standing in your way, like a bird that can fly above it all.

Wisdom

The yoga of expressing your creativity can be a quest inward. This journey is a way to get to know your nuances and quirks; they make you amazing and unique, more yourself than anyone else.

Learning to embrace these gifts can help you factor in your other traits (good and bad). Moving through all your parts with the same sort of balance you work for in your yoga practice will help you become the whole you.

Wisdom is defined as "the quality of having experience, knowledge, and good judgment; the quality of being wise."

The wisdom of yoga is to be without judgment or self-doubt as you become aware of the nature and causes of your thoughts, feelings, and actions in an exploration of who you are. This allows you to be who you are within and outside some of the factors (internal and external) that try to define you.

Wisdom emerges from exploring who you know and understand yourself to be at various moments of your life—highs, lows, when someone notices you, when you notice someone. Wisdom is being all right with the truth that you will never know everything completely, but can become empowered enough to shoot your best arrow.

The workings of the world are much larger and more intricately layered than you can ever fully conceive, but if your eyes are open to you within the space you are creating, you will catch the most beautiful glimpses of all the possibilities.

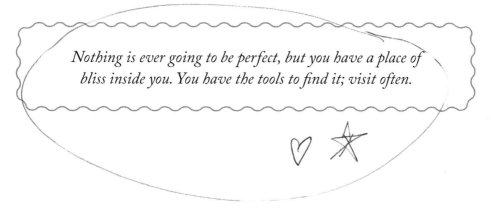

Nothing is ever going to be perfect, but you have a place of bliss inside you. You have the tools to find it; visit often.

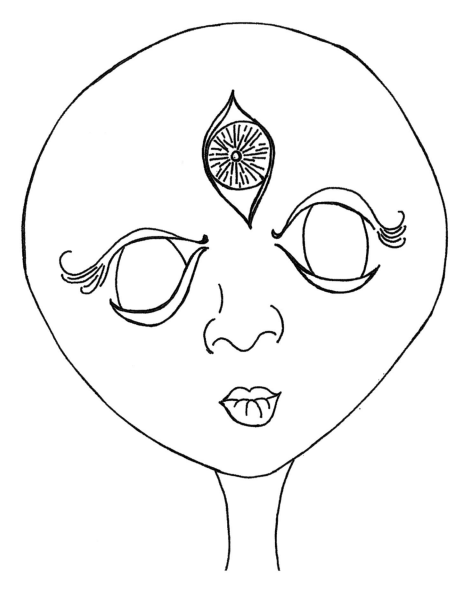

Look at your face in the mirror.
Close your eyes and begin to sense your third
eye at the center of your forehead.
Your "wisdom eye" is a source of power.

Intention

Yoga is a practice of intention. Intentions focus on the present moment; they are positive thoughts you use to guide your efforts. Your thoughts have power, your words carry meaning, and your actions have consequences creating small and large ripples in the cosmic pond. When you set an intention it should be positive and make you feel good about your role and efforts in what you are experiencing. Setting an intention as you practice yoga can help you find your right place in this large space.

The cosmic pond encompasses your *dharma* (the right way of living for you) and the effects of your *karma* (how your intentions and actions create your present moment, which have been influenced by your past, and will contribute to your future). Imagine everybody's stuff (past, present, and future) swirling around in a vast reservoir representing all peoples' energy at, and during, all times.

Your intentions (and intentioning) can change your world. They can affect how you view "*you,*" other people, places, things, issues that effect our universe, as well as your purpose in the spaces you inhabit.

Our affirmation for setting intentions is: *If I look with positive, energetic eyes, my world will be brighter. If all I can see is negativity, then it may become my experience.*

Your intentions (your efforts) might be constant and unchanging or morph and change hourly, daily:

  * Make a regular time and space to set and examine your efforts: to observe, to maintain, to reset, to live, to revisit, to revise, and practice.

  * Use your wisdom eye and the unique space you carry in your head and heart to get in touch with what is true for you.

  * Make your efforts and thoughts match what you want to happen in the present moment.

Your intentions, like your yoga poses, are fluid markers for who you are and who you want to become, as well as what you believe to be true right now, leaving space for you to redraw or rewrite or reshape their meaning when you see or feel something you can do to help yourself and the world around you.

My intentions are my own creation.

Setting My Intentions

Setting an intention is like making a goal, but not in the sense of achieving. Intentions are more about states of being:

* choosing the way you think about a dilemma or troubling situation

* choosing the way you will act in response to your triggers

* choosing the way you feel at any given moment.

My intention is my wave in the cosmic pond.
Waves have tremendous strength.

Intentioning is making an (affirmative) truth that guides you in your best direction in the present moment, your right now. *My intentions are powerful.* Here are examples of how you can go about identifying an intention that you believe in and will manifest through your thoughts, words, and actions.

   Intention: I want to feel gratitude—thankful in this moment though that might not be what the universe outside me is telling me (to feel).

   Intention: I want to send good energy to a story I heard today that makes me sad [insert a story about someone else's circumstances that you wish you could help]. I want to send energy toward a good situation I experienced or heard about today (this builds more positive energy); right here, right now.

My Intentions

Intention:

~~My Intention~~ My intention for starting School is to be focused. ♡

Intention:

My intention for ~~track is to work hard~~ my runs is to breathe and stay relaxed.

Intention:

My intention fo NaNoRiMo is to stay on track.

My Mantra

Create a mantra (your prayer or positive affirmation) that you tell yourself so often it becomes your truth. Your mantra is like an intention, always with you and OK to repeat over and over to yourself. It will probably take you a few tries to find just the right mantra. You might have several that you interchange, depending on how you are feeling and what you are experiencing. Give yourself room to feel into the best mantra for you, knowing that the only thing constant is change.

Mantra:

I am in this moment and focusing on what is here in front of me. ♡

Mantra:

~~I am doing my best and~~ ~~benefit~~
My actions acheeve maximum ~~results~~
with minimum ~~effort~~
effort ("I am in flow")

Mantra:

I am ~~sample~~ using this plan to complete this good and right.

~~~~~~~~~~~~~~~~~~~~~~~~~~~~~~~

CHAPTER 2

Practicing Yoga

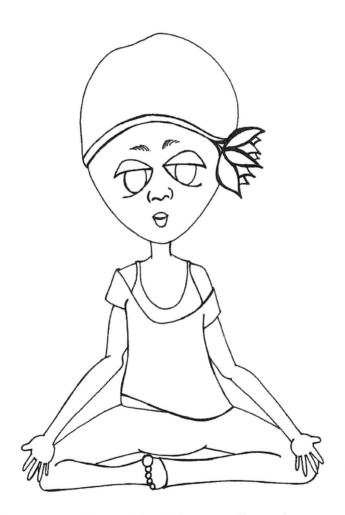

Throughout Yoga Girls' Club, you will see the names
and shapes of yoga postures in English and Sanskrit
(the ancient Indic language of their origin).

What is Yoga?

Yoga is a practice of getting to know you, inside and out, through movement, breath, and focusing within. There are no rules, no right or wrong, just you exploring who you are.

Your *dharma* and *karma* underlie the philosophy of yoga. These ideas can help you to identify your life purpose as well as uncover clues about how and why you exist in particular circumstances.

Dharma is intentional. It is about discovering your purpose in this place by doing what you love, for yourself and for others, while causing the least amount of harm possible to other creatures and beings. *Karma* is the result of your thoughts, words, and actions, and other stuff beyond your control—the cosmic pond. Combined, your *dharma* and *karma* are reflections of your character; they can impact your destiny.

Yoga is the practice of being the best person you can be in each moment, forgiving yourself for things you wish you had done differently, and trying to do better or make things righter the next time around. It involves intentionally setting the goal to be present and consciously aware each time you bring your journey to your yoga space.

Some days you might be a fierce warrior, having fought hard for who you most are that day. You might feel as if you are split into a million fragments, scattered all over the place—a *Comfortable Seat* might be a position or concept your mind and body need to embrace. You might need to sink in *Downward-Facing Dog* and feel: *I am home here.* You may need to hover above your world in a *Plank*. Let's move forward and decide today.

Do not stress about trying to do every pose right or the best way possible (every time is the first time), but listen to what seems most right 'r you and those you care about moment to moment. Stuff happens. 'Jur yoga practice is:

* I want to get to know myself in the midst of all the stuff.

* I will learn as I live my life.

* I am the key to unlocking the depths of who I am.

* I am becoming…

Observe how you feel as you explore the yoga postures, breathing exercises, and meditation techniques. As you practice, intentionally look at your life as you are experiencing it.

Use your practice to charge your body, your brain, you.

Ask Yourself

How do I feel in this moment?

Am I happy?

What are my gifts?

How can I stretch myself?

Can I see my light?

Can I feel my light?

Can I shine my light?

Can I turn my light back on if forces I do not control extinguish it?

Do I like me?

Can I grow my gifts?

This is your journey. Who you are in this moment is more powerful than your past actions, your *karma* (which you cannot control).

You can (even now) regulate your emotions by forgiving yourself and sending energy toward the change you desire.

Then you choose to move on.

Your future is *intentioning* your *dharma*: finding what you love, doing what you love, and serving as only you can in the cosmos.

* I am me.

* I am whole.

* I am creative.

* I am filled with light.

* My light and energy are important to the universe.

Petals of Yoga

Patanjali Maharishi, a sage (a wise person), gathered rules or guidelines for how we could be our best selves as we live in the world. They are called the eight limbs of yoga and are part of a larger text, the *Yoga Sutra*. The limbs are observations that contain general truths about ways of being, and principles and techniques to be practiced over time to bring your body, mind, and spirit into a personal state of harmony.

Let's visualize the eight limbs of yoga as seven petals of a flower, revolving around a center of bright happiness. The petals offer ways to work toward being happy with who you are and being happy with your actions (what you do) in the world. Together, the petals create a beautiful and unique blossom that reflects you. It takes a balance of all of the petals and their center, your center, to experience the peace and joy inside of you, which can bring you in harmony with what is occurring outside you, where change happens constantly, even as you blink your eyes.

Start exploring the petal that speaks to something inside you. Practice that petal every day, and over time the other petals will fall in place. Practicing the petals of yoga takes time. Give yourself a non-judgmental space where you can try them out. This space might be on your mat, in your space where you practice yoga; it might be quiet, you might like calm music without words—take time to create this space. Then begin your practice and notice how your process grows. You are making good energy, creating rich soil around you because you are a flower blooming in time and space, connected to everything, yet free to be *you*.

Let's talk about the seven petals of yoga and their center…

The first petal, the *Yamas*, describe the ways you should try to interact with others. The *Yamas* are:

* *Ahimsa*—stepping softly in the world without causing harm.

* *Satya*—being honest and truthful.

* *Asteya*—not taking or stealing what is not yours.

* *Brahmacharya*—figuring out what is and is not for you, sometimes practicing self-control, others times letting your entire self free to experience and be the full expression of you (inside and out).

* *Aparigraha*—not hoarding or holding too tightly or collecting a lot of what you do not need.

The second petal, the *Niyamas*, focus on the ways you should be with yourself. The *Niyamas* are:

* *Saucha*—cleaning your body and personal space, while trying to think mostly good thoughts.

* *Santosha*—being aware of the joy deep inside you.

* *Tapas*—holding yourself responsible for doing what you know you should do (right, wrong, based on your truth).

* *Svadhyaya*—study yourself; spend time getting to know yourself and where you fit in the world by exploring what you like and do not like, and why.

* *Ishvara Pranidhana*—acknowledging that there is a power greater than you.

Asanas, the yoga postures, form the third petal. When you practice the yoga postures, not only do you do them with your body, you experience them and feel them in your mind and in your emotions. The postures can help you figure out if you feel sad, alone, happy, or full, as they prepare your inner space, *you inside you*, your center, to be calm, quiet, clear, creative… You are making a space where your best self can emerge and grow.

The fourth petal, *Pranayama*, works with your breath to quiet your mind and center your focus. A *Pranayama* practice is a powerful way to harness your energy and how it flows. By itself, the word prana refers to life force, the spirit or energy of life that gives you strength, movement, zest, sparkle, and the shine inside you. When you learn to guide your breath, your prana becomes stronger.

The fifth petal, *Pratyahara*, means paying attention to what is happening inside you.

The sixth petal, *Dharana*, means focusing your attention on a single point. By building your ability to concentrate on one thing, you can control your moods, your reactions, your actions, and change the balance between how you see the good parts of your day clearly from the bad.

The seventh petal, *Dhyana*, invites you to think deeply about what you are focusing on. Where your attention goes, your energy follows. When you experience *Dhyana*, you can meditate (be still and calm inside) with a clear, quiet, focused mind. And when your mind is in its best state, you might discover that those things you think about a lot, or are trying to figure out, become clearer… Whether you are at a crossroads where you don't know what to do next, making big decisions, thinking about where you fit in your family, in school… You might be able to figure things out by sitting with yourself and opening the space to "see" yourself—what you want, where you are, where you want to go, now, then. Here (in *Dhyana*), you might learn to like yourself, to love yourself and others, as you live and breathe in your home, community, and in the world.

As you spend time with the petals of your yoga flower, you are working, every day, on who you are, who you want to become. When you like who you are, when you are happy with the person you are just because you are "you," then you are dwelling in *Samadhi*, the shining space in the middle of the flower.

As you move from the petals to Samadhi, the center of the flower, you are moving from the things and forces outside of you to your center, where peace and joy and calm, and the creating spirit of the universe live in you. You are tapping into the good in you; your most powerful, happy, and complete "you."

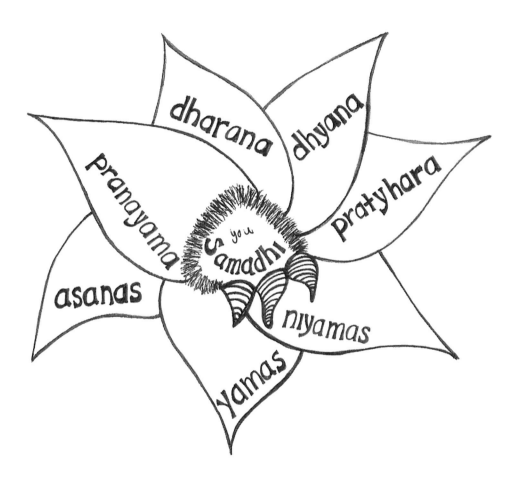

CHAPTER 3

Breathing

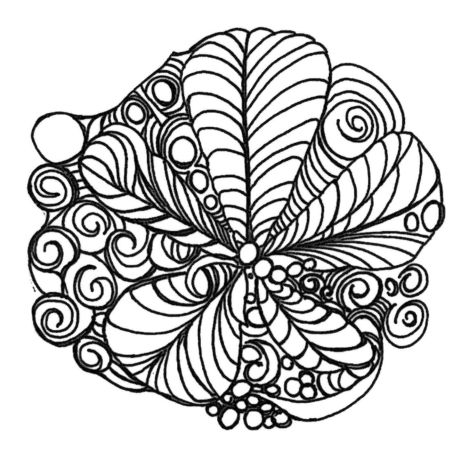

Be yourself with your every breath.

Three-Part Breathing

For *Three-Part Breathing*, you will divide your breath into three parts as you breathe into your belly (the bottom of your lungs), into your rib cage (the middle of your lungs), and into your chest (the very top of your lungs). This is a calming breath that you can practice anyplace, anytime.

Inflate your belly with breath, count: *one*, *two*. With the same breath, expand your rib cage, count: *one*, *two*. Same breath, fill your chest with breath, count: *one*, *two*. Hold your breath in for a count of two.

Breathe out from the space of your chest, count: *one*, *two*. Same breath, knit your ribs together as they empty of air, count: *one*, *two*. Same breath, deflate your belly as you empty your lungs completely: *one*, *two*. Hold your breath out for a count of two.

Swell and deflate your belly like a balloon, feel your ribs expand and contract like an accordion, and experience your chest rising and falling like waves in the sea for nine rounds of breathing.

You might:

* record how you feel before practicing *Three-Part Breathing*

* record how you feel after clearing your lungs, head, nose, and throat

* consider what triggers your stress and what triggers your calm.

Ocean Breathing

Deepen your inhalations and exhalations for *Ocean Breathing*. Fill your belly, ribs, and chest with breath just like in *Three-Part Breathing*. Begin to make your exhalations longer and your inhalations deeper, warming your stomach-core.

When you breathe like the ocean, your breath sounds like the waves. This breath, through your nose, is the one you will want to practice while doing yoga postures.

Open your mouth; imagine you are fogging a glass window with your breath. As you mist the glass, make the sound "HAAAA." Breathe in the same sound, "HAAAA." Do this a few times, getting a feel for the flow of your breath through your mouth and throat. Close your mouth (the glass is adequately fogged). Feel how your breath moving in your throat sounds the inner strings of your vocal chords. Equal parts in with your breath, equals parts out.

Inhale and exhale through your nose, as you narrow and expand the passageway of your throat. Listen to your breath moving, feel your breath guiding your movements; focus on your breath, allow it to quiet your mind and fuel your movements.

Do this breath by itself for nine rounds and incorporate it into the shape of your yoga postures. Your movements, expansion, and contraction will tell you how to breathe.

Alternate Nostril Breathing

For *Alternate Nostril Breathing* you will breathe into the left side of your nose, hold your breath in center, and then breathe out of the right side of your nose, alternately inhaling and exhaling through each side of your nose.

It is not as complicated as it might sound. Try to notice how your breath is flowing, and for a few minutes, before you start, just flow with it. This breath balances your sides, your emotions, your chaos as it brings you into balance, your center.

Place the index and middle finger of your RIGHT hand between your eyebrows. Gently press the space between your eyebrows with the tips of your fingers. This is your third eye *chakra*. It is said that your wisdom resides here. Extend your ring and pinkie finger to the LEFT and your thumb out to the RIGHT.

Exhale completely.

Close your RIGHT nostril by pressing your thumb gently on it. Breathe in through the LEFT side of your nose.

Use your ring finger to close your LEFT nostril, hold your breath in center. Focus on your air. Lift your thumb, opening your RIGHT nostril, and breathe out.

Inhale through your RIGHT nostril. Still holding your LEFT nostril, close your RIGHT nostril. Hold—focus on your *prana*, the life-giving force of your breath. Open your LEFT nostril and exhale.

Inhale through your LEFT nostril. Close both nostrils. Open your RIGHT nostril and exhale.

Continue, left to right nine times. Complete this breath by exhaling out of the LEFT side of your nose (creating balance because you took your first inhalation through this nostril).

Feel your breath moving equally through both sides of your nose as you begin to breathe normally.

CHAPTER 4

Flowing Postures

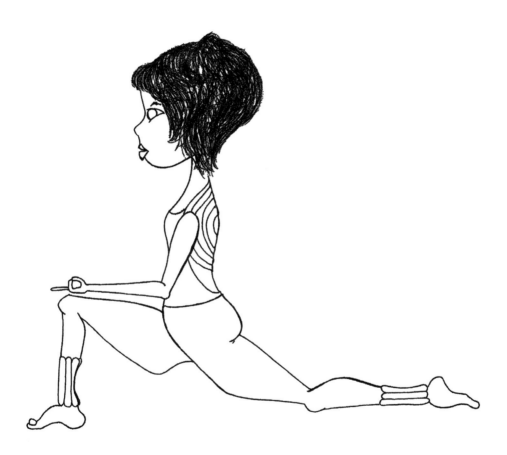

Feel into the poses, give them color and shape. As you
move within and through them, listen to your body.

Cat and Cow
Marjaryasana and *Bitilasana*

Start on your hands and knees. Place your wrists and elbows under your shoulders, splay your fingers wide (starfish hands), and position your knees hip distance apart under your hips. Line your knees up with your hips, so the space between them may be small. Stack your joints and limbs in this way each time you come to this pose.

Relax the top of your feet to the earth and begin to feel strength building in your belly as you draw your navel gently in toward your spine.

Breathe out, arching your back like an angry cat as your navel continues to curve up into your spine; feel your head and your hips hanging heavily toward the earth in *Cat* pose.

Breathe in, intentionally lift your head, lower your belly, and lift your hips toward the sky, moving into *Cow* pose; feel your spine gently arching up at your tailbone and the top of your head. This slope forms the bottom of a strong and gentle U, you.

Move with the natural flow of your breath, breathing out to arch into *Cat*, breathing in to lengthen (slope) your back into *Cow*. Some days you may breathe in and out in the opposite direction; just breathe your breath and become aware of your own flow each time you practice.

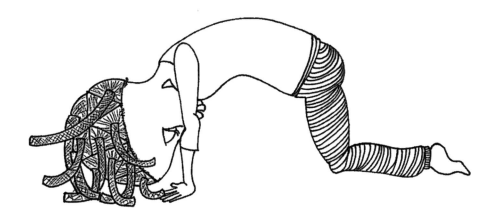

Cat

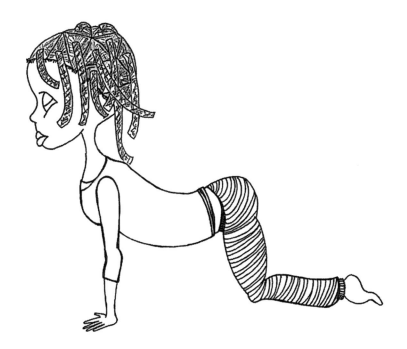

Cow

Spinal Balance

On your hands and knees, make sure your joints and limbs are stacked—arms directly under your shoulders, knees in line with your hips. Gently pull in your belly to support the length of your spine from your head to your hips. Make minor adjustments now and whenever you lose your alignment. Your poses are fluid creations, but as you flow through them keep your joints safe.

Level out your shoulders and hips from the top of your head to the base of your spine. Your back is sturdy like a table; *think about a vase of your favorite flowers resting on the stability of your back*. Stare down at the mat directly under your head.

Breathe in, extending your RIGHT leg back behind you, and point your toes downward. Reach your LEFT hand forward, turning your thumb upward as you look beyond it. Lift your gaze to slowly focus on the horizon before you. *See your ability to handle anything it holds*.

Breathe out. Intentionally lower your gaze, and place your hand and knee back on the surface below you. Start again, feeling the ground beneath your palms, knees, and tops of feet; inhale and exhale.

Let's move to the other side. Breathe in, extend your LEFT leg back, flexing into your foot; feel stable and reach your RIGHT hand forward—thumb up. Check the view on this side. Breathe out, connecting back to earth.

Continue to alternate your sides until your belly feels warm and strong. Flow from side to side with the movement of your breath. Keep your belly firm and your spine long, strengthening your stomach-core. Find your rhythm as you extend your arm and leg forward and back. At times, when you come to this position, your bottom knee might be wobbly, your arm tired. It's OK; feel into your strength and ability to reach.

At that moment when you feel balanced, *notice what makes the difference*. Store this in your mind and revisit this awareness whenever you need to find balance in your day, your tasks, and your moods. If you can find your place in *Spinal Balance*, think of how much power you have on two feet.

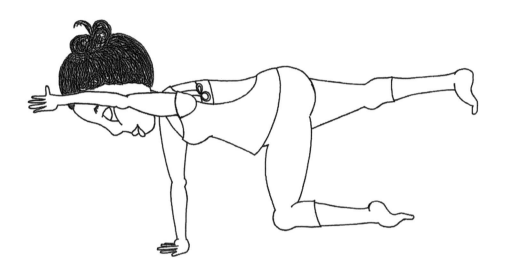

Spinal Balance

Mountain
Tadasana

Stand tall with your feet about hip distance apart—make fists with your hands, bend over, and place them between your feet—this is "about hip distance" when the insides of your feet touch your pinkie fingers. Parallel the inner lines of your feet to each other like railroad tracks running into the distance.

Point your second toes forward and line your heels up behind them. Ground your feet into the earth. Lift your toes up toward your ankles; feel how this pushes the base of your big and little toes into the floor. Press down these two points and feel into the center of your heels. Lower your toes one at a time: *you can access this wave of energy even inside the most uncomfortable shoes, or situations, if you think about these tiny movements or see them in your mind.*

From the solid base of your feet, feel your entire body lengthening up toward the sky. Bend your knees softly, a tiny micro-bend, so that you are not locking your knee joints. Relax your thighs and butt, feel them hanging heavy; gently pull your belly in—bringing your navel toward your back. Lift your heart up and out as you roll your shoulders back and down. *Feel into this sensation.*

Your arms are hanging heavy from your shoulders; turn your palms forward, and open your fingers wide. Feel length in your neck as your chin parallels the earth and the crown of your head reaches toward the sky.

Now scan your body from your feet up. *Do you feel grounded or ready to fly?*

Like a mountain, feel strong and immovable in *Mountain* pose. Breathe full and deep. When you feel your most grounded, begin to imagine the possibility of climbing mountaintops, and leaving your footprints behind as you gather what you need from each precipice, with each breath, moving closer to you and the gifts you bring to and will continuously give this world.

Remember to breathe; it helps.

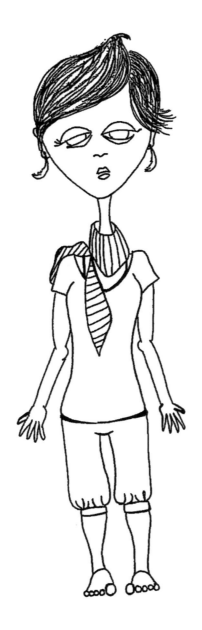

Mountain

Upward Salute
Urdhva Hastasana

From *Mountain* pose, breathe in, sweeping your arms out to the side and up toward the sky; connect your palms overhead. Feel into this space.

Breathe out; float your connected palms down to your heart center. This position for your hands is *Anjali Mudra*—a gesture of offering yourself to this moment. *Mudras* are symbolic gestures designed to awaken spiritual energies in your body.

Inhale; release your hands down by your side. *Take in the fullness (even if it feels like emptiness) of what you are feeling*.

Glide your hands up from your sides again; feel your arms floating upward like the wings of a bird, soft and flexible, powerful and strong, as your palms connect over your head like two old friends.

Imagine yourself reaching for, catching, and then drawing a fluttering butterfly (or whatever you find beautiful) down to your heart for a moment, and then releasing it. This movement is gentle, yet strong; close your eyes and feel yourself moving freely in space.

Exhale. Draw your hands down in front of the space of your heart.

What is floating by? If it is good, memorize how it looks, feels, and tastes. What do you hear inside you? Is it bad? Acknowledge its presence, push it away, move through it carefully, with growing confidence that you leave it behind.

Do this seven times (an auspicious, divine number); each time your hands pass your heart, think: *I am reaching for my dreams. I am holding them. I have all I need, already, inside of me.*

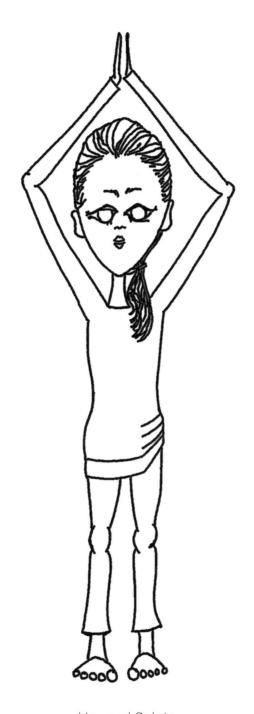

Upward Salute

Chair
Utkatasana

From *Upward Salute*, breathe out, sweep your arms down by your sides and then forward and up as you lower your hips into an imaginary chair. Just like in *Mountain*, your feet are parallel to each other and as you bend your knees they move in the same direction as your toes—straight in front of you.

Your knees are stacked over your toes; your thighs form a 90-degree (right) angle with your legs. Each body is different; work toward your best interpretation of these perpendicular lines each time you sink into your *Chair* pose; tweak and adjust by listening to what your body tells you each time you practice.

Breathe in, press down through your feet to rise and stand tall. Sweep your hands skyward into *Upward Salute*.

Continue this flow with your breath, sitting into *Chair* as you exhale, standing tall each time you inhale. *How does it feel to sink and rise? How much effort does it take? What is your natural flow? Do you feel the connection between your movements and your breath?*

Feel your heart lifting as your tailbone drops low. You are more upright than leaning forward. Gently engage your belly—draw it up and in—to support the length of your spine and prevent a scoop in your back.

What do you need as you sit in this powerful seat? Do you feel light, heavy, or in between? What colors do you think of when you ground, when you lift?

Do this several times. If your arms get tired, connect your fingertips and palms in front of your heart in *Anjali Mudra*, harnessing your own energy, or rest your hands on the tops of your thighs as you flow in and out of your seat using the strength of your legs and the lightness your breath creates in your body.

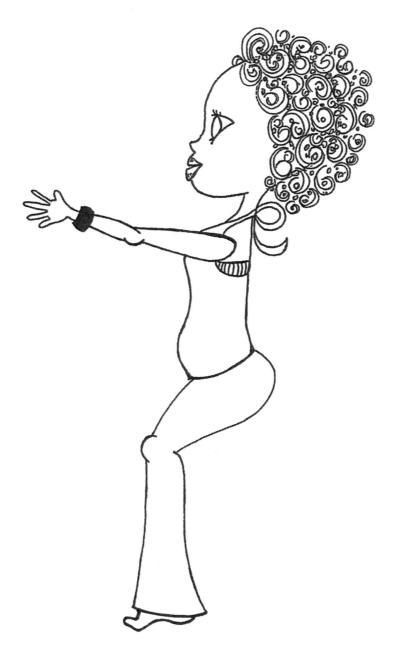

Chair

Forward Fold
Uttanasana

From *Upward Salute*, breathe out as you open your arms wide, bend at your waist, turn your palms down and lower, like a swan diving to the earth. Bend your knees enough so that your hands connect to the floor; your fingertips might barely touch the surface beneath you or your palms might be flat to the earth. Feel as though you are hinging from your hips, which allows your back to remain long as you fold.

Relax the muscles in your neck. Gently shake your head a few times, up and down, for *yes*, and then side to side, for *no. Grow strong in both motions. Your character is connected to your ability to decide between yes and no.*

Inhale. Expand your arms out to the side like wings, turn your palms up as you lift your torso and float your arms overhead. Exhale, fold, bending your knees, and hinge forward from your hips. *You are not falling, but choosing to surrender to this moment. This is a moment of freedom and control.*

Look toward your belly as you relax your neck and let your head hang—nod your head *yes*, and shake it *no* again, until you can find a still place to let go. Then just hang. *Giving yourself a few minutes not to decide anything is also essential to cultivating who you are.*

Flow between *Forward Fold* and *Upward Salute* for three rounds of breath, maintaining a slight bend in your knees and length in your spine, as you listen to, observe, and watch your breath. Begin to feel into all of your parts as you lift and lower, gathering and releasing who you are. Here, you might see some of the things you need to hold tightly and others you need to release.

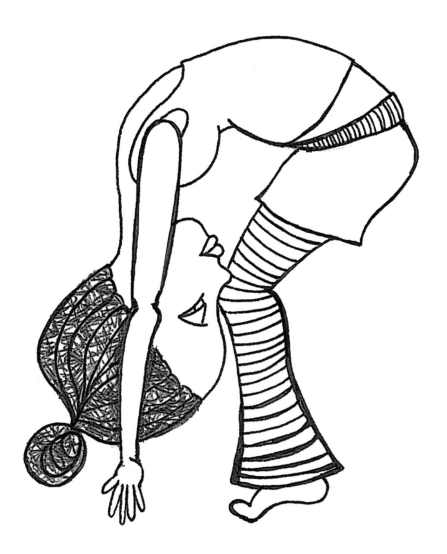

Forward Fold

Crescent Lunge
Anjaneyasana

From *Forward Fold*, hands flat on the ground or strong in your tepee shape, step your RIGHT foot back long as you bend into your front knee. Stack your front knee straight over your ankle—make sure your big toe is visible beyond your knee. Give yourself enough space between your feet so your back heel can lift directly over your toes.

Elongate your back leg by pressing out through your heel (almost as if the back of your foot is pressing on a wall behind you—your toes are still down). Leave the tiniest bend in your knee to prevent locking it. Bend your front knee deeply, working your thigh parallel to earth, creating a 90-degree angle with your front leg.

Feel strong in your belly as your hips sink downward and your torso lifts up. Draw your tailbone toward the earth, lengthening your spine.

To vary your *Crescent Lunge*, you can keep your hands on the ground—make a tent with your fingers, or use yoga blocks if it is uncomfortable to keep your hands that far down. Yoga blocks allow you to build the floor up to your body's natural point for doing a posture. *Your source of power is different from that of another person. One of your intentions can be to grow strong in your postures, aware of and honoring your strengths.*

When you feel strong in the base of your *Crescent Lunge*, breathe in and lift your shoulders over your hips. Rest your hands on your front thigh, keep them there, or place your palms together in *Anjali Mudra* in front of your heart, or reach your arms up to the sky, working the bend out of your elbows.

Hold for a complete inhalation and a full exhalation. *Feel into this place. What do you see and feel here?* Exhale.

Place your hands back to earth or your blocks. Step your RIGHT foot forward into *Forward Fold*. As you inhale, float your LEFT foot back, rebuilding *Crescent Lunge* on your other side.

After you get strong and find your center of balance in *Crescent Lunge* on both sides, return to your *Forward Fold*. Release your hands to the ground, stack them under your shoulders; starfish your fingers, flatten them, and press firmly on the ground. Step your feet back one at a time—

side by side, facing forward, keeping your hip distance. Lower your knees down, lining them up under your hips. Rest on all fours—your hands and knees. *Crescent Lunge is a posture of balance, power, and strength.*

Your point of balance is one of your gifts.

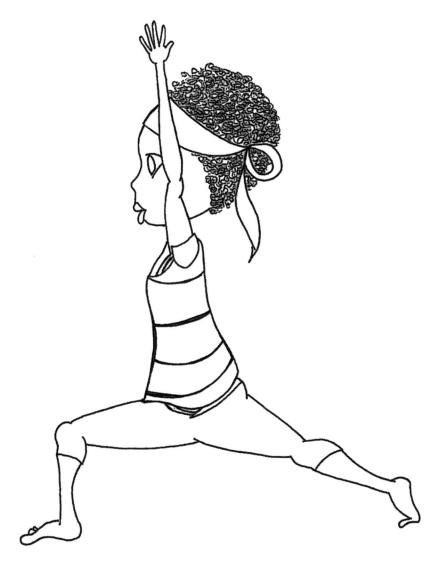

Crescent Lunge

Child's Pose
Balasana

From your hands and knees, breathe out and float your hips back to rest on or above your heels as you lengthen your arms out straight in front of you. Reach farther than you think you can, starfishing your fingers; your elbows are lifted.

If you need more space for your stomach or your hips, widen your knees toward the edges of your mat; feel your big toes touching behind you. Sink into the space this creates in your hips. Each time you practice, it's different, so tweak with every breath, and make adjustments natural to your body. Surrender. Rest your forehead on the ground or your block. Melt into *Child's Pose, Balasana—can you see balance leading this Sanskrit word?*

Melt your shoulders, deepen your breath, and turn your attention inside, to *you*. Take as many breaths as you like here. Relax into this posture. Feel restful and supported. As you get comfortable, you might slide your hands down by your feet—turn your palms up to take pressure or stress out of your shoulders, or stack your hands one on top of the other and rest your head on the pillow of your hands (full of your strength and your good intentions).

* *What do you feel right here, right now?*

* *Are you low to the earth or are you riding the planets?*

* *Are you resting on a cloud or still thinking about what you should be doing?*

Here—try to release everything you're holding—now in *Child's Pose*.

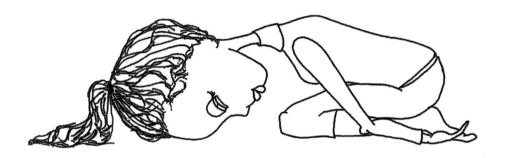

Child's Pose

Downward-Facing Dog
Adho Mukha Svanasana

From *Child's Pose*, reach forward through your fingers, lengthening your arms, and make a strong connection to the surface beneath you. Tuck your toes under behind you, feel the bottom of each toe touching the ground. Begin to press down into your hands (starfish fingers) and the base of your feet—though your heels are lifted. Draw in the pit of your belly, lift the center of your body up, let your navel pull you toward the sky. You are making a pyramid. Your hands and feet are the base, your arms and legs the sides, your tailbone the vertex, the highest point, soaring above civilization since 2630 BC when construction began on the earliest-known Egyptian pyramid. *Think of all the good intentions, energy, and dreams you have stored inside of you.*

Try this to make your *Downward-Facing Dog* feel even better: press down through the inner edge of your hands (still spread wide with your index fingers forward, index finger and thumb side flattening the pad of your hands out to your little fingers), bringing length and space into your wrists. Bend your knees slightly to draw more of your weight into your legs and out of your upper body.

Drop through your heels (feel them reaching for the floor), elongating the backs of your legs. This shift of weight back and down allows you to ease even more pressure off your wrists and out of your shoulders, which leaves a natural space for your neck and head to line up with your arms.

Feel your arms, legs, and back lengthening in *Downward-Facing Dog*. Relax into your own strength here, for three rounds of breath. Maintain a soft bend in your knees and elbows when they are holding you up. Each time you breathe out, relax deeper into the posture.

Every time you land in *Downward-Facing Dog*, think of it as home. It is a position of rest and restoration, an inversion, which energizes your brain because your head is lower than your heart.

✳ *What do you feel as you settle into your* Downward-Facing Dog?

✳ *Are your thoughts clearer, your imaginings more vivid when your head is below your heart?*

✳ *What colors do you see?*

✳ *Is it the floor beneath you or something more vast?*

Transitions are smoother if you are solid in your home base.
How you move from pose to pose, from side to side,
is incredibly important in yoga, as in life.

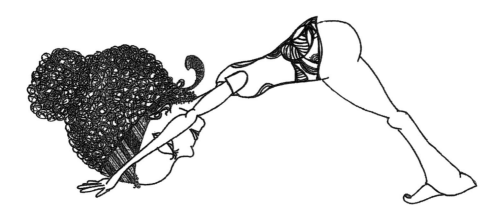

Downward-Facing Dog

Flow Your Flow

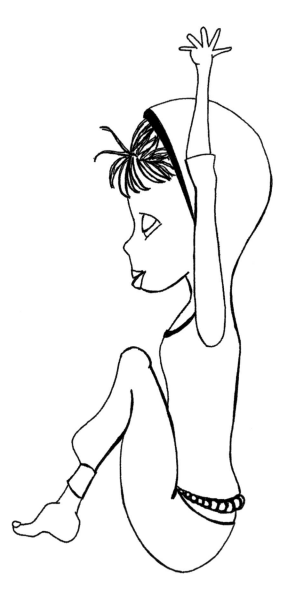

You may experience a fluid flow all at once; you might not. You have to spend time exploring your body and how it feels as you move through the following three postures. When you use your inhalations and exhalations to guide these postures between holding your *Downward-Facing Dog* pose, it is called a *Vinyasa*. *Vinyasa* means to place your body in a special way, guided by your breath.

Plank

From *Downward-Facing Dog*, inhale and roll your shoulders forward to meet your wrists in a strong vertical, stacked line (wrists and elbows under your shoulders). Your heels rise above your toes. When you feel solid, begin to feel into the length of your body.

Press back through your heels to straighten your legs more (but try not to lock your knees). Pull in through your belly to activate your core (some say this is your powerhouse); lift and engage the space behind your heart and look to the earth slightly in front of you.

This is like a high push-up. *Do you feel yourself getting stronger? You are.* Maintain for three rounds of breath.

In moments where you need to make your *Plank* a little more kind, lower your knees down gently (keep your feet tucked and active). Create a straight line from your knee joints to the crown of your head. This is *Knee Down Plank*.

Your elbows are snug to your torso; work to keep them in this position; they point back toward your waist and feet as you lower your torso to the next posture, *Four-Limbed Staff*.

Some days a *Knee Down Plank* might feel better than one with your knees lifted. Try not to be stuck in doing things one way. Switch it up by intentionally listening to what your body tells you it needs on any given day, in a given movement.

Plank builds strength and endurance; it can also help you change your perspective.

❊ *If a lot of chaos surrounds you when you stand on your feet, what happens to the air, to your thoughts, to your energy when you come close to a surface where you're not likely to fall, a surface that is charged with years of survival to energize your roots?*

❊ *What happens inside you as you hover in your* Plank, *lower to* Four-Limbed Staff, *rise to* Plank *again, lower to* Four-Limbed Staff *another time before you glide to* Baby Cobra *or* Upward-Facing Dog *and finally float up into* Downward-Facing Dog—*then rise and walk forward into your next moment?*

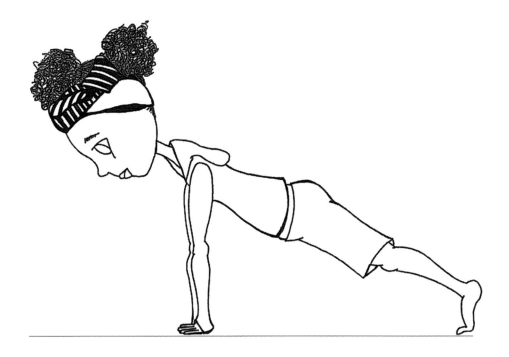

Plank

Knee Down Four-Limbed Staff
Knee Down Chataranga Dandasana

Child's Pose transitions to your *Knee Down Plank*. *Knee Down Four-Limbed Staff*, a variation of *Four-Limbed Staff*, begins here so you can flow into *Baby Cobra*.

From your *Child's Pose* move to *Knee Down Plank*, and breathe in, bringing more length and space into your body (your arms are stacked under your shoulders); place your gaze on a steady point on the horizon in front of you (your neck is long, supporting the lift in your head); lift the center of your heart, feel your chest strong.

Breathe out and begin to bend your elbows back toward your chest and waist, keep them in close to your sides as you lower your torso halfway down. Hover your torso above the earth like a helicopter flying level and low.

Breathe in and lower your hips and belly and heart all the way down to the earth, keeping your back straight. Now, flatten the tops of your feet on your mat, press down through your thighs, and draw in through your belly.

Get ready to float your palms above the earth for *Baby Cobra* (see the next pose).

You are building a series of movements; keep going.

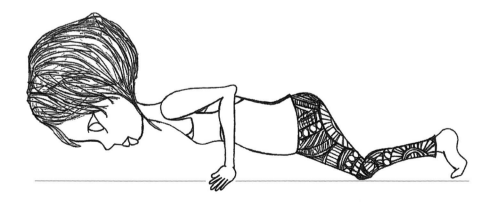

Knee Down Four-Limbed Staff

Baby Cobra
Bhujangasana

If you are moving through your *Knee Down Four-Limbed Staff* (a *Four-Limbed Staff* variation), you are going to lower your belly to earth in *Baby Cobra*. Do *Baby Cobra* until you strengthen your arms and get used to opening your shoulders and lengthening the muscles in your lower back, then move on to *Upward-Facing Dog*. Choose how you want to layer them into your practice. Some days *Baby Cobra* will feel better in your back, arms, and shoulders; other days *Upward-Facing Dog*. Listen to your body: it will tell you which is best.

From *Knee Down Four-Limbed Staff*, hover your torso above the ground, release the tuck of your toes by flattening onto the tops of your feet. Exhale and lower your belly to the surface below you in a solid piece (arms close to your chest, pressing back toward your hips—your chest, shoulders, and forehead come down to the mat at the same time) as you begin lifting your heart and extending your gaze a few feet in front of you.

Check in: make sure your palms are level with your chest; intentionally tighten your belly (pull your navel in toward your spine) to support this pose. Lift your gaze, shoulders, chest, heart, and hands up (off your mat) like a snake rising from its belly forward (except snakes don't have arms). Press the tops of your thighs and tops of your feet down, gently lifting your torso even higher into *Baby Cobra*. Here, with your hands free of weight and pressures, you might feel as if you are flying through time and space.

From *Baby Cobra* exhale and bring your hands back to earth (near your chest), and press into them. Keep your knees down and move your hips back to your heels in *Child's Pose*. Like *Downward-Facing Dog*, *Child's Pose* is a resting posture, another home. Feel into this stillness after all of the transitions you made through this flowing series. *How does the air feel around you? What else do you notice? Hear? See? Imagine? Right now, what do you think you can create?*

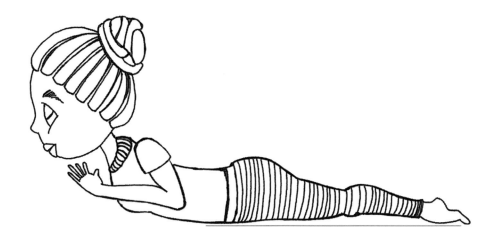

Baby Cobra

Four-Limbed Staff
Chataranga Dandasana

Four-Limbed Staff with knees lifted connects *Plank* to *Upward-Facing Dog*.

From *Plank*, keep your knees lifted, or you can place them down on your mat for the *Knee Down Four-Limbed Staff* variation you have been practicing. *You will know when you are ready. Your knees will stay up and your arms will feel strong as you hold your* Plank *above your mat. This might remind you of the high part of a push-up.*

In *Plank* (knees up) your toes are tucked. Press back through your heels, aligning them over your toes (straightening your legs with strength). Exhale, lower your body (head, neck, shoulders, and back in a solid, straight line)—halfway between where you were and the ground—by bending your elbows back (hug them into your rib cage) as your whole body hovers above the earth.

This is your *Four-Limbed Staff*—your body is in a straight line running parallel to the surface below you.

Keep your hands (with starfish fingers) firm and grounded as you inhale; release the tuck of your toes, placing the tops of your feet (one at a time) to your mat; keep your knees lifted and your hips off the earth as your heart and head float skyward into *Upward-Facing Dog* (see the next pose).

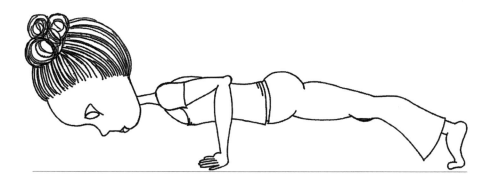

Four-Limbed Staff

Upward-Facing Dog
Urdhva Mukha Svanasana

If you are moving from *Four-Limbed Staff* and floating into *Upward-Facing Dog*, you will be holding your body up by your feet and the stacked strength of the palms of your hands (your thighs and legs are lifted).

From *Four-Limbed Staff* with your knees lifted and your body parallel to the earth, release the tuck of your toes and gently place the tops of your feet (flip them down) to the earth.

Press down through the tops of your feet and the strength of your hands and arms to lift your legs, knees, thighs, hips, lower back, and belly (keep your stomach-core strong) above the floor into *Upward-Facing Dog*.

From *Upward-Facing Dog*, breathe out, tuck your toes under your feet again (feel the bottom of each toe touching the ground). Get sturdy, pull your navel in toward your hips, rise skyward into your *Downward-Facing Dog* (strong starfish hands, feet hip distance, tummy engaged—you are a pyramid that can weather any storm).

Downward-Facing Dog should feel like a good home—your safe harbor. Rest. Feel new.

Notice:

* *What do you feel in this pose?*

* *What did you sense during your movement?*

* *Did you see a dark night or a dawning day or something else?*

* *What colors did you see: yellow, orange, blue, or some combination the world has not discovered yet?*

* *What did you discover about you?*

* *Was your breathing rhythmic, shallow?*

* *Did your perspective expand or contract with movement?*

* *What are you connected to as you explore your thoughts?*

A Mantra Filled with Your Possibilities

I am created for movement, I am always in motion.

I can decide if this rhythm should be slow or fast.

I can regulate my actions, reactions, and decisions.

I am right here, right now.

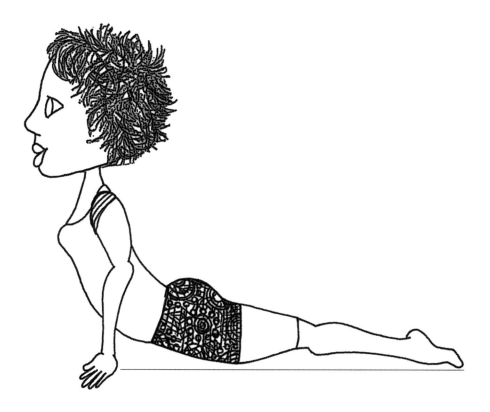

Upward-Facing Dog

Vinyasa

Vinyasa means to place in a special way, and in the midst of a yoga practice it often decribes the linking of the following postures with your breath:

Vinyasa

Downward-Facing Dog

Plank

Four-Limbed Staff

Upward-Facing Dog

Downward-Facing Dog

Your inhalations and exhalations give each movement in this series life. You flow through a *Vinyasa* to progress through a cycle of your movements the way midnight leads to the morning sun and lunchtime and nightfall to a new moon. *How will you fuel these cycles? How will you intentionally control your* Vinyasa—*placing yourself and moving—through the energy pulsing through you, from you, and around you?*

On days when a *Vinyasa* feels challenging, work up to it in stages. Begin to build strength by entering your flow with the following postures:

Vinyasa Variation

Child's Pose

Knee Down Plank

Knee Down Four-Limbed Staff

Baby Cobra

Child's Pose

Move through your day with awareness of where you place your body and how you breathe your breath.

Synchronize your breath with your movements.

Practice means doing yoga over and over, not necessarily seeking perfection, but to discover more of you.

* *Move mindfully through transitions.*

* *Move with purpose.*

* *Move with kindness (to yourself and others) and strength.*

* *Feel your feet firm beneath you.*

Being Me

I am powerful.

I am fluid on this journey.

I have more to learn about myself today.

Breathing with Intention

Here are your options for the *Vinyasa Flow*. Both sides of the table strengthen your arms and stomach-core. The left side of the chart can feel more challenging while the right side can seem more inviting. Pick the variation that feels best for you the day you practice.

Placing the flow of your breath…

Vinyasa	Breath	Vinyasa Variation
Downward-Facing Dog	Exhale	*Child's Pose*
Plank	Inhale	*Knee Down Plank*
Four-Limbed Staff	Exhale	*Knee Down Four-Limbed Staff*
Upward-Facing Dog	Inhale	*Baby Cobra*
Downward-Facing Dog	Exhale	*Child's Pose*

*You can bring some measure of control to your
world by controlling your breathing.
Then you can see new avenues, or the best, even
if it is the familiar route, open to you.*

Sun Salutations
Surya Namaskar

Sun Salutations combine all of the flowing postures into a fluid series of movements guided by the flow of your breath, *prana*. You can move through *Sun Salutations* slowly, taking a couple of breaths in each posture, or you can move through them vigorously, taking one breath in each posture before flowing to the next.

Whether your pace is slow or fast, take the time to feel your body's alignment, stacking your poses from your base (feet, toes, hands—whatever is touching the earth) up. As you press down, feel your energy lifting you up. Say to yourself: *Press down to lift up.*

A complete round of *Sun Salutations* begins with your RIGHT leg leading, stepping back at the beginning of your salute to the sun and forward with your RIGHT foot at the end for another *Crescent Lunge*, and continues as you seek balance by letting your LEFT leg lead, stepping back and forward with your LEFT foot for *Crescent Lunge*.

Our sides, like our five senses, are full of rich layers that affect the way our body works. Strenghtening your sides keeps your body in shape, full of energy, noticing, and alert in helping you make sense of your world.

Sun Salutations

Sun Salutation	Breath	Sun Salutation Variation
Mountain	Exhale	*Mountain*
Upward Salute—swan-dive your arms down, starfish hands on earth	Inhale	*Upward Salute*—swan-dive your arms down, starfish hands on earth
Forward Fold—step RIGHT foot back, keep your knee high, press out through the center of your lifted heel, toes stay on earth	Exhale	*Forward Fold*—starfish hands stay on earth, step RIGHT foot back and lower knee to earth

cont.

Sun Salutation	Breath	Sun Salutation Variation
Crescent Lunge—reach your hands up, long spine, then starfish hands on earth, step LEFT foot back to meet RIGHT foot	Inhale	*Low Lunge*—reach your hands up, long spine, then starfish hands on earth, then slide LEFT knee back to meet RIGHT knee, and sit hips toward heels
Downward-Facing Dog	Exhale	*Child's Pose*
Plank	Inhale	*Knee Down Plank*
Four-Limbed Staff	Exhale	*Knee Down Four-Limbed Staff*
Upward-Facing Dog	Inhale	*Baby Cobra*
Downward-Facing Dog—step your RIGHT foot forward between your hands, bend into your RIGHT knee	Exhale	*Child's Pose*—starfish hands stay to earth, reach long through your arms, rise and slide your RIGHT foot forward between your hands
Crescent Lunge—reach hands up, long spine, then starfish hands to earth and step your LEFT foot forward to meet your RIGHT foot	Inhale	*Low Lunge*—reach your hands up, long spine, then starfish hands on earth, tuck the toes of your LEFT (back) foot under, raising your knee from earth and step your LEFT foot forward to meet your RIGHT foot
Forward Fold—hang heavy	Exhale	*Forward Fold*—hang heavy
Upward Salute—reverse swan-dive your arms up, starfish hands reach high to sky	Inhale	*Upward Salute*—reverse swan-dive your arms up, starfish hands reach high to sky
Mountain—bring your palms together and down to your heart	Exhale	*Mountain*—bring your palms together and down to your heart

Repeat the flow on your LEFT side—step back for Crescent Lunge *with your LEFT foot and after your journey step forward into* Crescent Lunge *with your LEFT foot.*

> *My conscious breath, movements, and thoughts*
> *contribute to the cosmic pond.*

Sun Salutations are especially good for:

* *greeting the sun of a new day—a new moment*

* *making a new beginning at any time in your day*

* *feeling the sun's warmth and remembering that you are in its reach*

* *energy*

* *blooming*

* *connecting to a source of power larger than you*

* *creating the space to set an intention (a personal design, that benefits you or your community, to direct your mind toward so you can begin to live into it)*

* *fueling your steps*

* *affecting/effecting your actions*

* *moving with purpose*

* *shining a light on the dreams that came to you in the night*

* *adding to your inner glow*

* *sending good energy to others*

* *sending good breaths into the universe.*

CHAPTER 5

Standing Postures

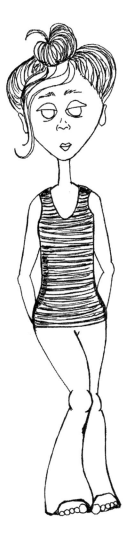

Feel your strength as you ground in who you
are and reach out into the universe.

Lateral Flexion
Ardha Chandrasana

Upward Salute with both hands reaching toward the sky, exhale and place your RIGHT hand down by your side. Bend gently as you try to touch the earth with your fingers as your top arm reaches higher (the LEFT one).

Press down through both of your feet equally; feel the center of your body rise as if weightless. This creates vertical length on both sides of your torso as you reach and give from your center. Try to relax your shoulders and lift your heart as your arms reach in opposite directions.

Hold for three rounds of breath as your gaze, your *dristhi*, moves to a place that steadies you and lengthens your neck.

Inhale, floating your torso to center as your hands meet overhead in *Upward Salute*.

Exhale, reach your LEFT hand to earth as you keep your lifted arm skyward (the RIGHT one). Hold for three rounds of breath on this side. Lift and lengthen, focus your awareness up and down both sides of your torso.

Inhale, *Upward Salute*, exhale and bring your hands down together in front of your heart in *Anjali Mudra*.

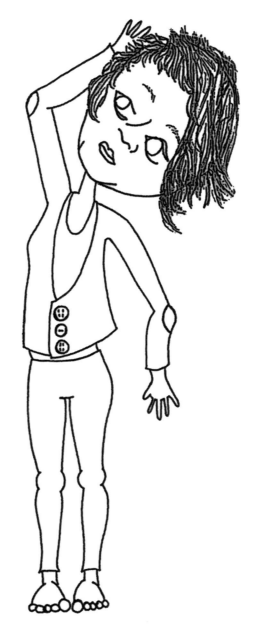

Lateral Flexion

Warrior II
Virabhadrasana II

From *Crescent Lunge* pose with hands touching the earth, and your RIGHT knee forward and your LEFT leg back (here, your heel is lifted over your toes), rotate your back heel down so that your whole back foot is flat to your mat, angle your toes slightly forward. Line up your feet so that if you extended a line from your front foot it would bisect the center of your back foot.

As the outer edge of your back foot connects to the floor, lift up through your inner arch (under your ankle). Your front knee is bending deeply over your ankle; gently open it out toward your pinkie toe. This is your *Warrior II* base.

Lift your shoulders over your hips, extending your RIGHT hand forward and your LEFT arm back so that your shoulders, heart, belly, and hips are open to the side. Draw a straight line with your arms above the earth, reaching dynamically front and back.

Drop your tailbone, as you lift the pit of the belly in and up toward the sky. Feel your back leg lengthening as your front knee bends (don't extend beyond your ankle—keep your joints safe by keeping them stacked). Look out over your front hand, softening into the pose.

Hold for three rounds of breath. As you exhale, cartwheel your hands to earth on either side of your front leg, raising your back heel over the base of your toes, returning to *Crescent Lunge* pose with hands down.

Step forward into *Forward Fold*. Hang for a breath or two before stepping your RIGHT leg back, bend your front LEFT knee. Rebuild *Warrior II* from your feet up on this side.

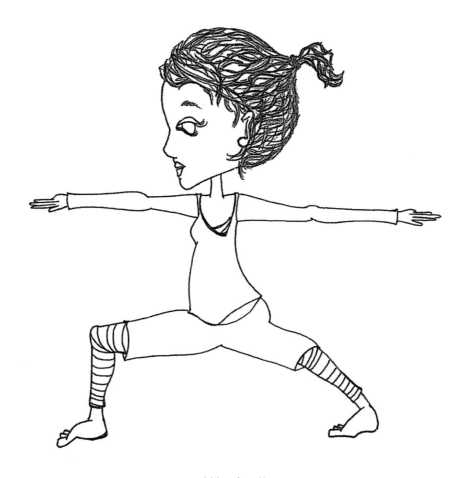

Warrior II

Triangle
Trikonasana

From *Warrior II*, with your RIGHT leg forward—deeply bending at your knee, with your back leg long, and your foot flat to the surface beneath you—inhale and straighten your front leg (keep a tiny bend in your knee to protect your knee joint).

Exhale, reaching as far forward as you can with your front hand; feel your torso long as you lower your hand to your leg wherever it lands without you folding forward. Everything is in one straight line as if you were a piece of bread in a toaster. Stack your shoulders as you reach your top arm up toward the sun, moon, or stars. Stack your hips as you press both feet firmly into your stability.

Feel as if your entire body is stacked, aligned, fluid, living, breathing in the right place at the right time. If your top arm gets tired, rest it on your hip. This is a bit of a twist; open your heart and your belly toward the sky of possibilities, finding a *dristhi* that is comfortable.

Inhale, lift your shoulders over your hips, stand tall.

Repeat *Triangle* on your opposite side; you can pivot on your heels facing the opposite way, rebuilding the pose from your feet up, or move through *Warrior II*; place both hands to earth and lift your heel for *Crescent Lunge* with hands to earth, step forward into your fold, then step your RIGHT foot back so your LEFT leg is forward.

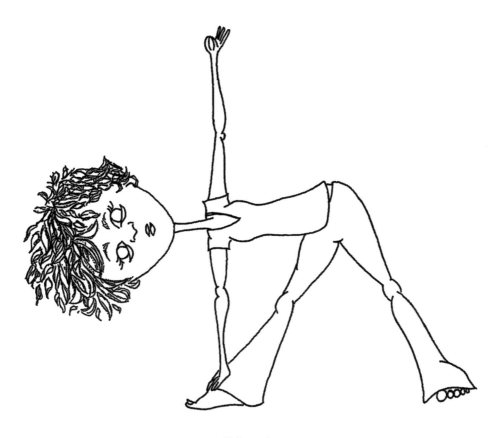

Triangle

Goddess Squat
Utkata Konasana

Come to the center of your mat, turn to face the side, step your feet out wide, make the inner edges of your feet parallel to each other, then turn your toes out at a diagonal.

Bend your knees, so that they stack right over your ankles; you may need to step your feet closer together or wider apart, so your ankles are right under your knees. Open your knees out wide toward your pinkie toes, creating a space for your tailbone to move down toward earth. You should feel this along the inner line of your legs.

Inhale, lift your arms up from your sides, connect your hands overhead. Exhale and bend your elbows—making your arms look like those of a cactus; feel them strong as your shoulders remain relaxed as you turn your palms up as if you were holding something precious in your palm. *Right here, right now, what are you holding?*

Feel your lightness and strength as you move your seat closer to earth. Breathe out, and bring even more length into your spine as you breathe in.

Be in *Goddess Squat* for a few rounds of breath. You are a goddess. Feel into your *Shakti*, your divine, feminine, and creative energy.

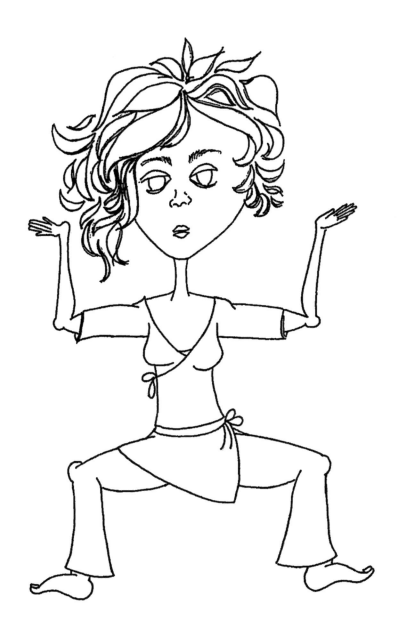

Goddess Squat

Standing Straddle
Prasarita Padottanasana

From *Goddess Squat*, inhale, straightening your legs, and reach your hands overhead into *Upward Salute*. Exhale, let your arms melt and hang heavily by your sides.

Parallel your feet to each other, pointing your toes forward and placing your heels directly behind them. Feel the outer edges of your feet grounded as your inner arches lift.

Inhale, reach your arms overhead. Exhale, fold forward from your hips as your arms reach out to the side and connect to earth at the bottom of your fold. Keep a little bend in your knees as you hang free.

Let any tension, tightness, and stress roll right off your back and out of your shoulders. Let your head hang heavy and feel your mind clearing. Breathe here, hold this space as long as it feels good.

When you are ready to come out of *Standing Straddle*, inhale, roll up from the base of your spine to the top of your head, slowly sweeping your arms overhead, then drawing them down to your heart. Check in, how are you feeling?

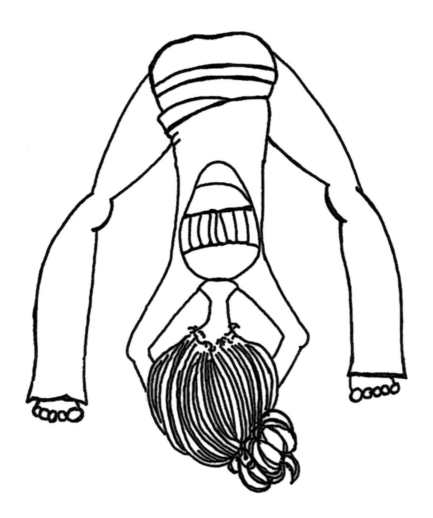

Standing Straddle

CHAPTER 6

Balancing Postures

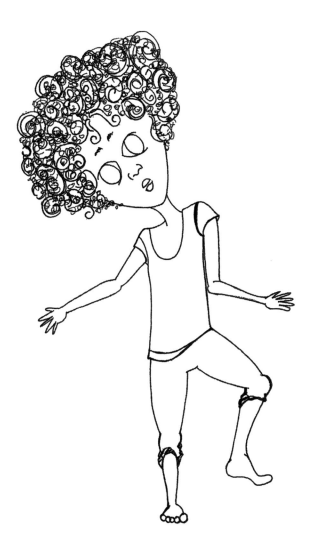

When the ground you are standing on is uneven, when it feels as if you are out of balance, when you feel discombobulated, it becomes even more important to be able to be in your center.

Tree
Vrksasana

From *Mountain* pose, bring your hands together in front of your heart in *Anjali Mudra*. Shift your weight onto your LEFT leg, energize your stomach muscles by engaging them, bend and lift your RIGHT knee up in front of your hip, and then out to the RIGHT side. Your navel and heart face forward as your knee opens to the side.

Place your foot at the inner line of your standing leg. Your heel can press to the inside of your ankle (toes touching earth) or your foot can come to your inner calf (below your knee) or reach down and place your foot on your inner thigh (above your knee). Make sure your whole foot is above or below your knee joint and then strongly press your foot into your leg and your leg back into your foot.

Lift your belly in and up, floating your heart high. Touch the tip of your tongue to the roof of your mouth, forming a *mudra* with your tongue. Like the hand *mudras* we have been doing, this movement is a symbolic gesture that helps you focus on your balance as it lifts you higher on your standing leg. As you inhale, you might extend your arms over your head, then grow branches with your arms or keep them in front of your heart. Say to yourself, *I am expansive and strong as I root into the earth and rise toward the sky.* Trees move in the wind. If you wobble, come back into the pose. Think strong and flexible.

If you extended your branches, bring your hands back toward each other overhead, exhale and lower your hands back to your heart space. Lower your foot. Ground. Relax, breathe into this moment. Build *Tree* standing on your RIGHT leg, lift your LEFT knee.

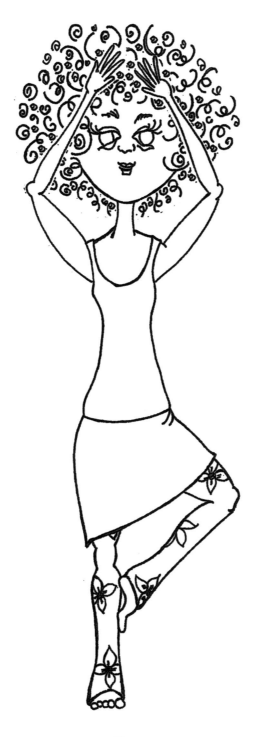

Tree

Dancer
Natarajasana

From *Mountain* pose, place your LEFT hand on your hip and bend your RIGHT knee. Reach out to the side with your RIGHT hand, turn your palm forward and point your thumb upward. With your RIGHT hand—your thumb is still pointing up and maybe touches the inside of your heel (so your shoulder is opening out and rolling down)—take hold of the inside of your RIGHT ankle. Bring your hips in line. Stand as straight as you can on one leg.

Keep your LEFT hand on your hip or extend your arm up over your head. Inhale, feel long from the bottom of your standing foot to the top of your head and out through your fingertips if you are reaching up. This is the beginning of *Dancer* pose.

Stay here (you're doing hard work), or, as you exhale, you might begin to fold forward from your hips. Reach your fingertips forward and up. Lift your heart and gaze to create an upward bend in your spine.

Inhale, float your torso up slowly, to stand with your shoulders over your hips. Release hold of your ankle with control. Relax both arms by your side. Stand tall and breathe deeply. When you are ready, work into *Dancer* with your LEFT hand holding the inside of your LEFT ankle. Dance gracefully, balancing through turbulence and victories. Can you hear your (inner) songs?

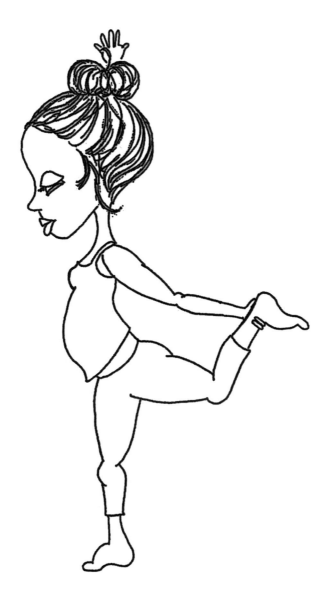

Dancer

Warrior III
Virabhadrasana III

From *Mountain* pose, swan-dive your torso parallel to the ground beneath you. Draw in your belly to support the length in your back. Reach your arms out from your shoulders like wings.

Shift your weight onto your LEFT leg, lift your RIGHT leg up behind you. As soon as your foot lifts from the ground, flex it by pressing out through your heel and pointing down through your toes (this energizes your leg).

Think about lifting your leg from behind your thigh (it's the heaviest, strongest part), level out through your leg and torso to create a straight line from the top of your head to the bottom of your foot. Steady your *dristhi* on a point that is not moving. Your hips are closed—facing in the same direction, the front of your RIGHT thigh is facing the ground.

To make *Warrior III* more challenging (if it is not enough already) reach your hands forward lengthening your arms—line your upper arms up with your ears. To make *Warrior III* less challenging, place your hands on your hips or to the floor or yoga blocks straight under your shoulders (*Supported Warrior*)—this is the best option if you find it difficult to balance today or if you feel uncomfortable on one leg.

Float light for a few rounds of breath. Warriors are powerful. Power is strongest when it's balanced and flexible. When you are ready to release, exhale into *Forward Fold*. Inhale, roll up. Exhale, dive parallel to the ground and lift your LEFT leg up behind you.

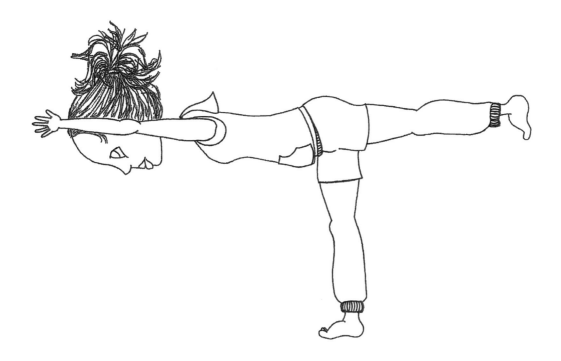

Warrior III

Balancing Half Moon
Ardha Chandrasana

For this *Balancing Half Moon*, you might want to use your yoga block. Place it in front of your mat. Stand tall in your *Mountain* pose.

Inhale your arms overhead, *Upward Salute*. Exhale, swan-dive to earth. Touch your fingertips to ground right under your shoulders (or place them on your blocks) so that your spine is lengthening forward and back. Feel the strength in your tummy, back, neck, and head. Inhale. Lift your RIGHT leg behind you (this is *Supported Warrior*).

Steady your *dristhi* and engage your core muscles as you place your RIGHT hand to your RIGHT hip. Keep your LEFT hand to the ground, lightly connecting your fingertips to the earth, or keep your hand squarely on your yoga block.

Stack your hips on top of each other—your hips and your shoulders are facing the right. Feel yourself opening to the side. Our sides are different, physically, mentally. What you feel and see on one side may be very different from the other. When things look unbalanced or fuzzy one way, try to find your balance in the other direction. Then figure out how they blend in the middle.

With steadiness, reach your RIGHT hand up to the sky, making a straight line from your bottom (grounded) hand across your shoulders up to your reaching fingers. Maybe you look up to the sky in line with your neck out to a horizon beyond the walls or space where you are practicing. A change of view can affect your sense of balance. Can you feel yourself floating light above the ground?

When you are ready to release, look down to the ground, bring your top hand to your hip, angling your hips toward earth. Both hands return to the ground or blocks, in *Supported Warrior*. Release your lifted leg beside your other foot. Take a few relaxing, deep breaths in your *Forward Fold*.

Repeat *Balancing Half Moon* on your other side. Lift your LEFT leg, create a firm base through your fingertips and standing leg. Gradually rise into your strength and lightness—you are half of the moon high in the night sky and some days.

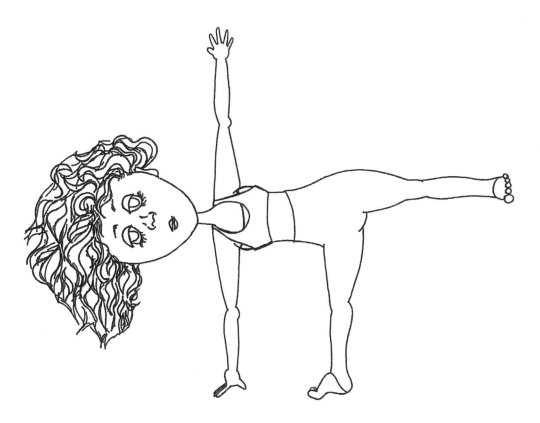

Balancing Half Moon

Bird of Paradise
Svarga Dvidasana

From *Standing Straddle,* with your feet out wide and parallel to each other and your hands strong on the earth under your shoulders, drape your belly over your thighs. You're going to thread your RIGHT arm under your RIGHT thigh. Try to place your shoulder behind your kneecap. Place your palm on the inside of your RIGHT knee; your thumb is up, your palm facing back behind you. Move it to the underside of your thigh as you inch your hand up the back of your thigh—your RIGHT knee has to bend slightly to make the space for your arm to reach toward you.

Wrap your LEFT arm around your back, palm facing out. With your RIGHT hand, try to take hold of your LEFT fingertips or maybe your LEFT wrist. This hold lands under the uppermost part of your RIGHT thigh. If your hands are far apart, use a yoga strap or scarf to fill the distance between your hands.

Now, with both arms wrapped around your RIGHT side, look down, establishing a steady *dristhi*. Heel-toe-heel-toe your LEFT foot toward the RIGHT foot so you can shift your weight onto your LEFT leg. Slowly, peel your RIGHT foot up from the floor.

Start to lift your torso as you maintain your hold on the RIGHT leg. As your shoulders come over your hips, begin to lift up in the space of your heart and get strong through your belly. From here you might straighten the leg you are holding; reach out through your big toe—you are a *Bird of Paradise*.

To land, bend your RIGHT knee if you straightened it, and float your foot back to earth with control; release the bind of your arms behind your back and thigh, and hang heavy in *Standing Straddle*.

When you are ready, repeat *Bird of Paradise* with your LEFT arm wrapping under your LEFT thigh and your RIGHT arm resting across your back. As your weight shifts onto your RIGHT leg, your LEFT leg and torso lift, floating up toward the sky.

Balance, like life, can be tricky. Some days you will soar right into this pose. Others you might wobble in it, or fall out once you're up. Be patient with yourself. Go back in… You can do this pose.

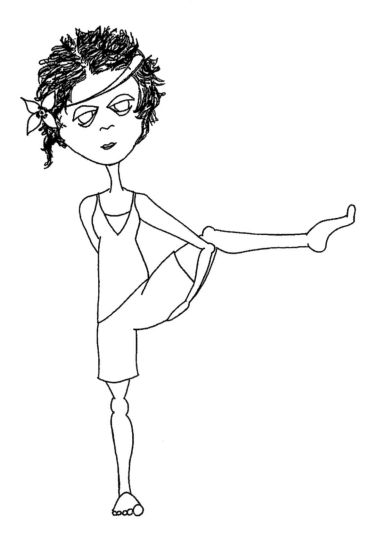

Bird of Paradise

CHAPTER 7

Sitting Postures

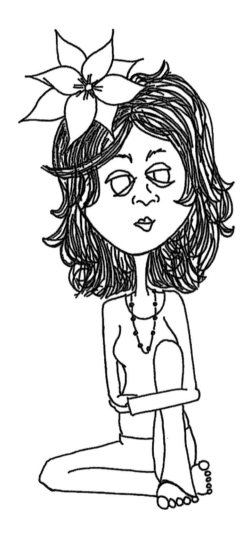

What does the ground, earth, world, universe, feel like beneath you?

Thunderbolt
Vajrasana

From your hands and knees, with the tops of your feet placed to ground, shift your hips back and take a seat on your heels. Feel your back long and strong enough to hold your dreams safely.

If your knees or any part of your legs hurt or if this position is uncomfortable, place a block between your feet and sit on it (a block has three heights, choose the one that is right for you), or put a blanket between the backs of your legs and the backs of your thighs to lessen the strain on your knees and the stretch of your quadriceps.

Rest your hands wherever they feel most comfortable—on your thighs, in *Anjali Mudra* (together in front of your heart), or you may want to place your palms over your heart. *Feel into your heartbeat and the movement of your breath.*

Close your eyes and listen to the rhythm of your breathing, drop into your space of calm.

I am here.

I am happy.

I am me, perfect and whole as I am.

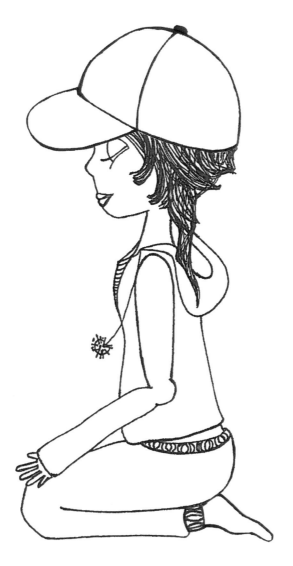

Thunderbolt

Butterfly
Baddha Konasana

Sitting with your hips on your mat or the stable surface beneath you, extend your legs in front of you and shake your legs gently to release all of the weight, stress, and responsibilities they carry around. Bend your knees, connect the bottoms of your feet and let your knees fall out and down toward earth.

Begin to press your tailbone down, lengthening your spine up like a flower rising out of the grass or a pond. Take hold of your ankles and relax your elbows on your thighs—your legs are heavy, open, with the outer edges supported by the ground. Fold over your legs, hang; or flutter through the air with the awareness that you are supported.

Breathe in. Exhale and roll your spine up bone by bone until your head is over your shoulders. Breathe out and melt your torso over your legs. Lift as you breathe in, fold as you breathe out, working with your breath. *Can you see your breath? Can you feel its power? Can you sense how it can work for or against you?* After a few rounds, hang heavy in the center. See (eyes open or closed) your heart in your mind and send energy and love and creativity to it. *Right here, right now, I feel…*

Hold this space as long as you like. When you are ready, inhale, roll up to a long, strong spine.

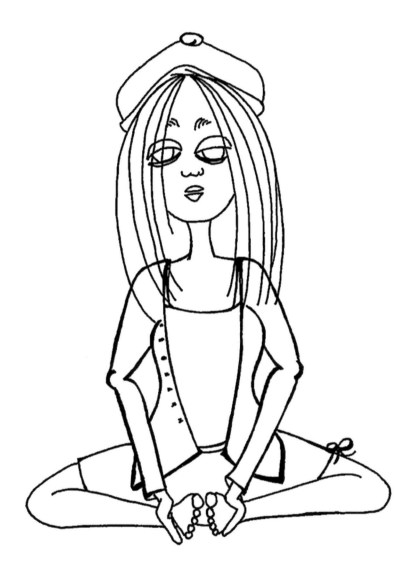

Butterfly

Boat
Navasana

From *Butterfly* pose, draw your knees up and in toward each other; place the bottoms of your feet firmly on the ground. Hold your legs behind your thighs and begin to tip your torso back so you come to balance on the bones at the bottom of your butt.

If balancing in *Boat* hurts your sitting bones or tailbone, place a blanket or some sort of thin, flat cushioning under you.

Feel as if a string is lifting your chest, softly pulling your heart upward. Engage through your belly muscles to support the length in your spine as you lean back. Tiptoe your feet close to your hips. Lift the back of your feet, just grazing the earth with your big toes. Shift back, keeping your balance—long-leaning back, engaged belly, supporting arms, and lift to a point where the weight of your legs is balancing the length in your torso. Strongly engage your core in the middle of your balanced V.

Keep your big toes to the earth, or begin to float your legs up— toes can hover above ground or your lower legs might come parallel to the earth—keep lifting your heart and *willing* lightness into your body. Balanced here, you might release hold of your legs and reach your hands forward toward your legs. Breathe. Imagine silk threads lifting your heart more, pulling your belly up and raising your feet. You might straighten your legs and lift your arms even higher to the stars. Sail on the support of your base. *Can you feel your center? Does you heart feel light?*

When you are ready to release *Boat*, exhale, take hold of your thighs, bend your knees, lower your feet toward the earth, touch down through your toes, releasing through all of the steps.

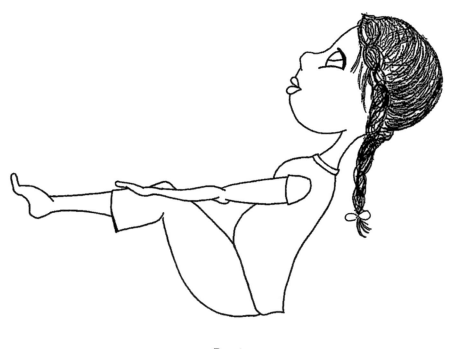

Boat

Table
Purvottanasana

Sitting on your mat, bend your knees and place your feet on the ground. Create hip-distance space between your feet. Press down through both feet: the base of your big toe, the base of your pinkie, and the center of your heel rooted strong on the ground.

Bring your hands behind you down on your mat. Place them under your wrists, angle your fingertips toward your feet, or out to the side if it is more comfortable for your wrists.

Flatten your palms and make sure your wrists are right under your shoulders. Feel stable and secure. From your belly (one of your power centers), float your chest, stomach, and hips skyward. Keep your head and neck in line with your spine. Lighten the front of your body as you press down through your hands and feet in *Table*.

Look to your belly as it rises and falls with your breath. As you breathe deeper, feel your belly expand with your breath, hold, watch and feel it empty as you exhale. Hold. Repeat. *Can you feel the center of your body light and heavy? As you watch the rhythm and presence of your breath, do you feel strong and stable, maybe even powerful? What does the view above you look like?*

Be present in *Table* for a few rounds of breath. Exhale, lower your hips to earth. Your arms are by your sides. Circle through your shoulders to release any pressure that might be there; first make circles up and back behind you, then circle your shoulders up and forward in front of you until you feel space in your upper back.

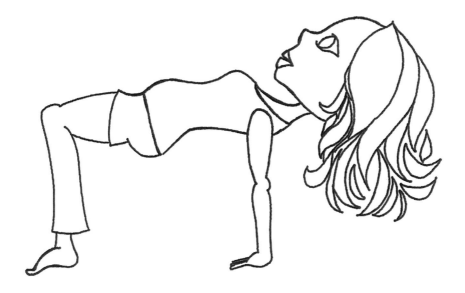

Table

Seated Spinal Twist
Ardha Matsyendrasana

With your hips on your mat and your spine long, extend your legs out in front of you. Rest your hands on the earth on either side of your hips. Your fingertips graze the floor, light as feathers, as you begin to draw in through your belly and lift up through your heart. Energize your legs by reaching your toes, vertical, back toward your torso.

Bend your RIGHT knee; make your foot flat against the floor about a fist's distance away from your LEFT knee. Weave your fingers together on the front of your RIGHT shin.

Inhale, lengthen your spine a bit more; exhale and twist from your belly, your heart, to gaze over your RIGHT knee in *Seated Spinal Twist*.

Each inhalation invites length and space up and down your spine. As your lungs empty of breath with each exhalation, you have more space to twist deeper to the side and maybe your gaze is on the world behind you. You might release your RIGHT hand behind you. Hold for several rounds of breath: in and out.

Inhale and bring your belly, heart, and gaze back to center. Exhale and extend both of your legs straight in front of you and fold over them. Breathe in to roll up from the base of your spine to the top of your head. Bend your LEFT knee, hold your shin; exhale and twist your belly, heart, and gaze over your LEFT knee in *Seated Spinal Twist*.

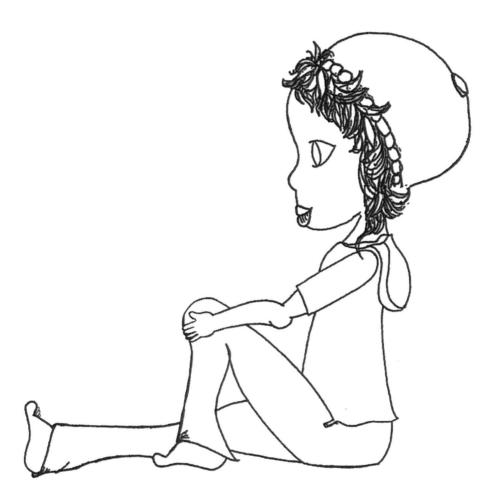

Seated Spinal Twist

Comfortable Seat
Sukhasana

Sitting on your mat, cross your legs in front of you. Draw the heel that is closest to your pelvis in a little closer, opening your knee wide, out to the side. Place your other heel in front of that one, so your ankles and shins do not cross, but one leg is resting in front of the other. This creates a triangular base for your *Comfortable Seat*.

Begin to lengthen your spine out of the base of your hips and legs. If it is difficult to lengthen your spine or you feel discomfort in your lower back, take your yoga block or pillow and sit on the forward edge of it, giving your seat a bit of lift (your butt is not completely on the block). It is also a good idea to prop your hips up if you feel any discomfort in your knees or hip joints.

Relax your shoulders. Connect your index finger and thumb together in *Jnana Mudra*, a hand gesture representing knowledge and wisdom of oneself. Your index finger represents the self you know yourself to be; your thumb symbolizes your infinite universal self that you are in the process of getting to know. Place your *mudras* in the same spot on your thighs or knees to create balance and harmony.

Close your eyes and deepen your breath, as you relax into your *Asana* (yoga pose).

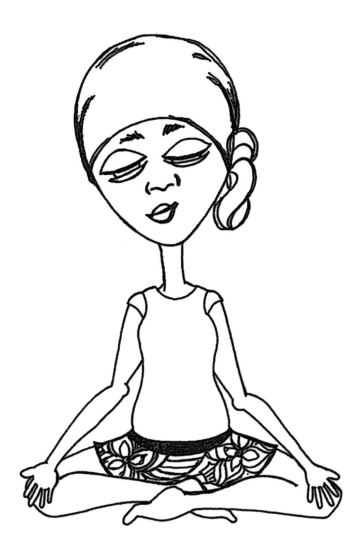

Comfortable Seat

CHAPTER 8

Inverting Postures

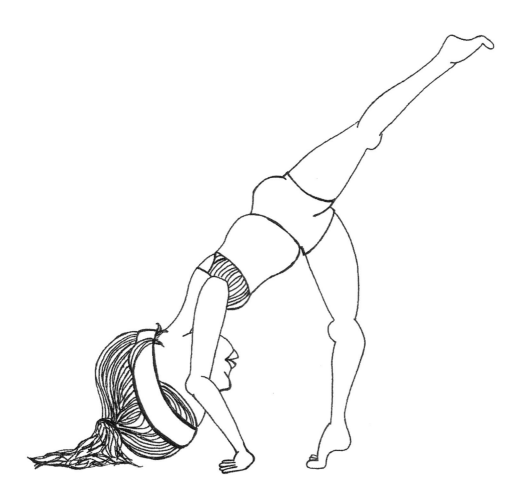

Remain steady, even, as your world turns upside down.

Bridge
Setu Bandha Sarvangasana

Lying on your back, bend your knees and walk your feet directly under them, hip distance apart. Feel the earth supporting the length of your back.

Keep your knees bent, feeling the ground down through your feet. Bring them close to your hips; keep a little bit of space between your knees. Make your feet parallel, lined up, with the sides of your mat. Place your arms down by your sides, palms to earth.

One of the secrets here: bring your feet as close as you can to your hands, which are reaching long toward your feet.

Broaden your shoulders and upper back. Begin to lift your heart upward. As you inhale, press down through your feet, your shoulders, and the backs of your arms and hands to float your hips upward.

Inhale. Press your knees forward, floating your hips higher. Imagine your breath as helium, lifting and relaxing the back of your body. Breathe into the altitude of your hips, feel lightness and spaciousness in your heart and hips supported by your breath. Watch your belly rising and falling. Keep lifting.

Hold for a few rounds of breath. When you are ready to release *Bridge*, melt your spine—upper back, middle back, lower back, then hips—down to earth.

Supported Bridge

To make this feel even better, place a block (a block has three heights—choose the one that feels comfortable) under the flat part of your lower back, then relax into its support. Resting on a block in Bridge takes most of the effort out of the posture. Lift your hips up from the block, place it to the side, and lower your spine down to earth.

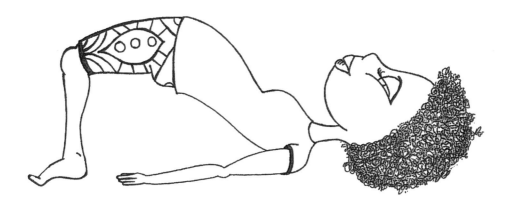

Bridge

Upward-Facing Bow
Urdhva Dhanurasana

Upward-Facing Bow pose is all about self-trust and waiting until you're ready to invert and lift like a spider; balancing upside down, you can raise your *Bridge* above a stable terrain. You might try this posture right away, or work yourself up to it. From *Bridge*, place your hands by your ears, pointing your fingertips toward your shoulders—palms down, spread like a starfish, and firm as you press against the ground and feel it pressing back. Draw your elbows in toward your head, stack them over your wrists. Keep your entire hand flat on the earth.

Exhale; press down through your hands and your feet to lift your body up. You might feel like an arching bow, an igloo, an overturned U. *How would you describe this sensation?* Take some moments to feel into the shape, positioning your hands where you feel strong and working your feet parallel to each other (these are tiny, gradual movements as if you are balancing a scale).

Inhale self-confidence and strength here. Let your head hang heavy but lifted above the surface under you. Feel your heart light. Hold for as long as you feel comfortable; breathe deeply.

To release *Upward-Facing Bow*, inhale, lift your chin toward your heart. Bend your arms slowly as you exhale. The back of your head softly touches ground first, then the rest of your spine lowers to ground from your neck down to your hips, vertebra by vertebra. Inhale when you are fully down; exhale and pull your knees to your chest, wrap your arms around your shins. Gently rock from side to side to massage the length of your back. Keep your head and hips grounded as you rock, releasing any tension in the middle of your body.

This inversion is sometime called *Wheel* pose.

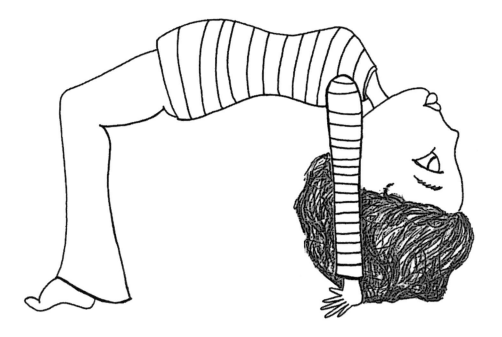

Upward-Facing Bow

Legs up the Wall
Viparita Karani

You can practice *Legs up the Wall* with or without a wall. With a wall, the posture is more restful because you do not have to hold your own legs up. Without the wall, you are using your core muscles to hold your legs up while actively stretching the backs of your legs as you press up through your heels to lengthen them.

For the wall variation, take a seat near an uncluttered wall. Connect your RIGHT shoulder and hip to the wall. Moving slowly, lower your head, torso, and top of your hips to the earth, simultaneously lifting and extending your legs straight up the wall. Your back is on the floor and your legs are reaching for the sky with the support of the wall. You might have to wiggle your hips closer to the wall until your seat and thighs are completely supported by its strength.

Check in here; it might be nice to open your legs wide, inviting an inner thigh stretch. You could try *Butterfly* up the wall, with your feet together and knees wide. Try any other variations of *Legs up the Wall* you can think of; just make sure your hips, thighs, legs, and feet are letting the wall carry their weight for a while. Let them rest here. Tell your back and arms and head to rest, too, accepting the earth's support.

Without the wall, lie down on your back, exhale and bend your knees, engage your belly muscles and lift your feet from the earth. Stack your bent knees over your hips. With your inhalation, extend your feet upward right over your knees. Flex your feet, drawing your toes back toward your heart—their flex is so active you could stand on the ceiling. As your legs lengthen up, relax your spine down, breathe deep and full into *Legs up the Wall*.

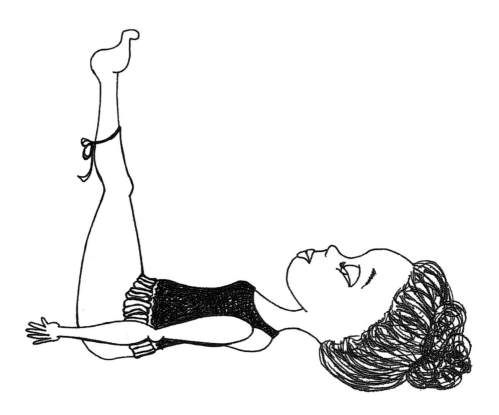

Legs up the Wall

CHAPTER 9

Reclining Postures

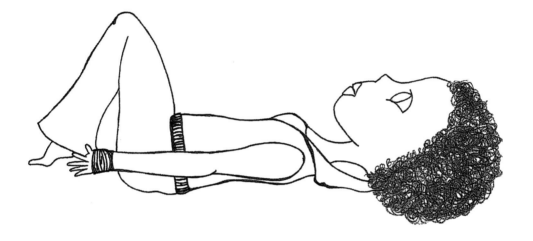

Relax your body, as you quiet your thoughts;
melt into the support of the earth.

Reclined Spinal Twist
Supta Parivartanasana

Lie on your back—flatten your torso and head to earth. Bend your knees, walk your feet close to your hips—maintain hip distance between them. Open your arms out wide to your sides, in line with your shoulders; turn your palms up, roll your shoulders back and down against your mat.

Breathe in to lengthen your spine. Breathe out, feel your body heavy on the ground supporting you. Press your feet firmly on the ground, pick up your hips, move them to the RIGHT side of your mat, and place them down.

Exhale; lower your knees all the way down to the LEFT. Keep both of your shoulders to earth and when you feel ready look out toward your RIGHT hand. Try to feel a twisting happening from the base of your tailbone to the crown of your head—seeing this image in your mind will help your body to feel the sensation. Let your legs relax and see if you can move your knees closer to your heart (this may be a little or a lot). Relax in *Reclined Spinal Twist* for several rounds of breath.

When you are ready, inhale and bring your legs and your head back to center—make this movement gentle and kind as your sides meet, new and old friends. Press your feet down on your mat and lift your hips, shift them to the LEFT side of your mat. Place your hips down and let your knees fall to the RIGHT side; feel supported on this side. After a few breaths, turn your gaze away from your legs and look toward your LEFT hand.

Let your inhale draw your knees back to center. Look at all of the possibilities above you, as you press through your feet and center your hips on the mat. Feel both shoulders heavy and solid on the earth. Breathe into the spaces *Reclined Spinal Twist* creates.

This movement can be slow and restorative as described above. Or you can keep your head, torso, arms, and feet on the ground (your knees are bent), and move your legs from side to side like windshield wipers in a rainstorm; exhaling as you move your knees to the side, inhaling as you move your knees to center.

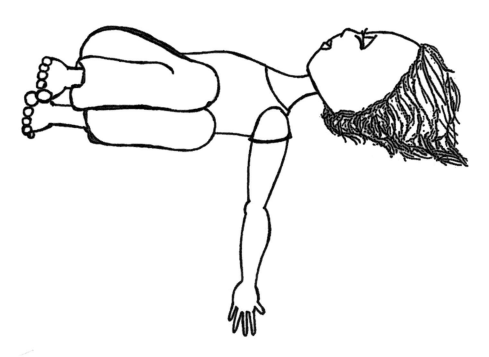

Reclined Spinal Twist

Happy Baby
Ananda Balasana

Lie on your back and draw your knees in toward your heart. Take a moment to be aware of how this feels. Connect your palms to the back of your thighs. Open your knees out wide to the sides of your torso, inviting your kneecaps to say hello to your armpits. Keep your back flat while you pull your legs wider and down toward the earth. Flex your feet, pressing their bottoms up toward the sky. With your back as flat as possible (from the back of your head down through your hips), rock gently from side to side in *Happy Baby*, giving your back a massage. This pose is also called *Dead Bug*.

As you maintain this deep bend in your knees, reach your hands up over your torso. Place your elbows alongside your knees and take hold of the outer edges of your feet. Even here, your back is flat to your mat. By holding your feet you're creating the opportunity for a deeper opening of your inner thighs and more compression of your intestines and stomach, which helps your food digest. Continue to rock gently if it feels good or find a still place in this pose.

Keep holding your feet or the back of your thighs in *Happy Baby*, extend your RIGHT leg out to the side. How does this movement feel on your LEFT side? Bend both knees, hugging them in toward your torso. Then straighten your LEFT leg out to the side. Notice how your RIGHT side changes.

Relax into this slow roll and rock from side to side. When you are ready, release hold of your legs, bring your knees together over your hips, and lower your feet to earth. Or for a challenge: with your knees in center over your hips, extend your legs to the sky. Hold for a few breaths, then lower your legs to the ground as you slowly count to ten.

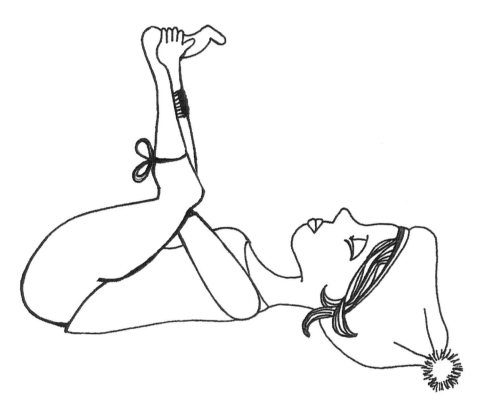

Happy Baby

Relaxation Pose
Savasana

For *Relaxation Pose*, flat on your back. Relax—breathe in slowly, breathe out just as slowly. You might create your own inhale thinking: *I am breathing in*; as you exhale: *I am breathing out*. Melt your body. Extend your RIGHT leg out to the right and your LEFT leg to its side. Rock your feet in and out a couple of times, letting them fall to stillness when they feel ready. Open your arms out to your sides and turn your palms up. Roll your shoulders back and down, nestling into the surface under you. Lift the space behind your heart. Inhale and exhale.

Relax your back. Allow your shoulders and the back of your head to rest, flat. Rock your head from side to side a couple of times, finding a comfortable place where it can rest. Relax your shoulders. Relax your belly. Feel your belly rising and falling with your breath. Make your mind as still as your body. When thoughts come to you, try to let them float by. Do you feel a sensation of peace? Your inside calm. Let this happen as it expands. This takes practice. Keep trying to let go in this awake-awareness. You are not sleeping.

When you are ready to re-energize your body from *Relaxation Pose*, take a deep breath in and release your breath out. Begin to wiggle your fingers and toes. Reach your arms long overhead and lengthen out through your legs, pointing out through your toes.

Bend your knees, taking a gentle roll to your right side; make a pillow of your bottom arm as you draw your knees in toward your heart. Bring something good and positive to mind; feel it in your heart, believe it in your mind, and plant it in your spirit.

Press down through your hands; lift yourself to your *Comfortable Seat*. Close your eyes for a moment; bring your hands together in front of your heart, bow your head toward them. Honor and acknowledge the creative spirit and the bright light within you.

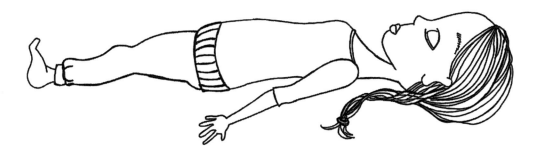

Relaxation Pose

CHAPTER 10

Yoga Flows

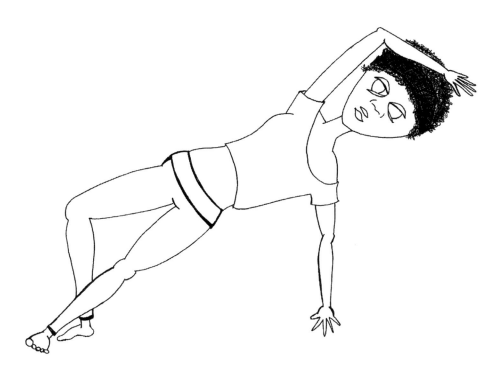

Explore the flows. See if moving this way changes your mood.
Do the flows change your point of view?

The yoga flow charts offer postures and breathing techniques you can do to change your mood and guide your energy.

As you practice, notice how you feel, how your body and mind respond to the movements and pauses… Remember, some of the postures will need to be done on both your right and left side.

Three of the flows include moments for meditation, being still and calm inside, which you can choose to include or try out later (you can read more about meditation in Chapter 11).

Creativity Flow

Flowing	*Child's Pose*
	Downward-Facing Dog
	Vinyasa or *Vinyasa Variation*
	Forward Fold

Standing	*Lateral Flexion*
	Warrior II
	Balancing Half Moon
	Triangle

Flowing	*Downward-Facing Dog*
	Vinyasa or *Vinyasa Variation*
	Chair

Balancing   *Bird of Paradise*

Sitting   *Boat*

                                           Seated Spinal Twist

                                           Butterfly

Inverting   *Upward-Facing Bow*

Reclining   *Happy Baby*

                                           Reclined Spinal Twist

                                           Relaxation Pose

Inspiration Flow

Breathing	Practice 7–9 rounds of *Ocean Breathing*—one inhalation and one exhalaion equals a round (p.40).

Flowing	*Mountain*
	Upward Salute
	Chair
	Forward Fold

Standing	*Crescent Lunge*
	Standing Straddle
	Goddess Squat

Balancing	*Dancer*

Flowing	*Spinal Balance*
	Cat and Cow

Sitting	*Thunderbolt*
	Table
	Boat
	Seated Spinal Twist
Reclining	*Happy Baby*
	Relaxation Pose
Sitting	*Comfortable Seat*
Meditating	*Sound the Quiet* (p.148)

Calm Down Flow

Reclining   *Relaxation Pose*

Sitting   *Butterfly*

Boat

Thunderbolt

Breathing   *Three-Part Breathing*

Standing   *Triangle*

Balancing   *Tree*

Meditating   *Move to Stillness* (p.149)

Inverting   *Legs up the Wall*

Reclining   *Happy Baby*

Relaxation Pose

Wake Up Flow

Sitting	*Comfortable Seat*

Breathing
Practice 3–9 rounds of *Alternate Nostril Breathing*—one inhalation with your LEFT nostril and one exhalation with your RIGHT nostril, plus one inhalation with your RIGHT nostril and one exhalation with your LEFT nostril equals a round (p. 41).

Standing
Lateral Flexion

Flowing
Sun Salutations

Standing
Crescent Lunge

Warrior II

Goddess

Balancing
Dancer

Warrior III

Tree

Sitting	*Table*
	Boat
	Butterfly
Inverting	*Bridge*
	Upward-Facing Bow
Reclining	*Reclined Spinal Twist*
	Happy Baby
Sitting	*Comfortable Seat*
Meditating	*Attune to Center* (p.148)

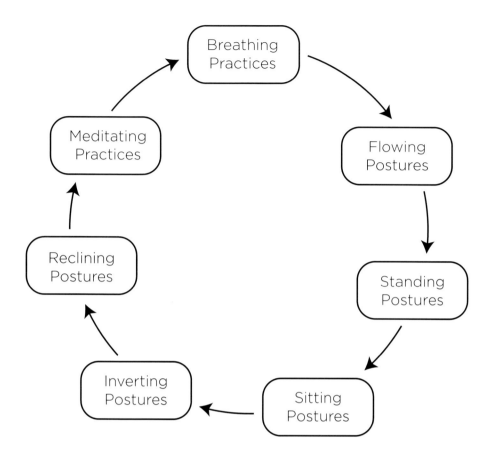

My Yoga Flows

Take some moments each day to feel into your flow, its up and downs and turnarounds—go with them, move through them, rather than pushing up against them. Honor your body's attempt to tell you what it needs from your practice.

Design your own yoga flows; place the postures in an order that speaks to you and your body.

Give your individual practices a name that reflects how they make you feel.

You are creating a library that reflects *you*—a book, your guide, your evolving strategies for moving through your world.

_____

_____

Breathing: _____

_____ Postures	
_____ Postures	
_____ Postures	
_____ Postures	
_____ Postures	

Meditating: _____

_____

_____

Breathing: _____	
_____ Postures	
_____ Postures	
_____ Postures	
_____ Postures	
_____ Postures	
Meditating: _____	

_____

_____

Breathing: _____	
_____ Postures	
_____ Postures	
_____ Postures	
_____ Postures	
_____ Postures	
Meditating: _____	

_____

_____

Breathing: _____	
_____ Postures	
_____ Postures	
_____ Postures	
_____ Postures	
_____ Postures	
Meditating: _____	

CHAPTER 11

Meditating

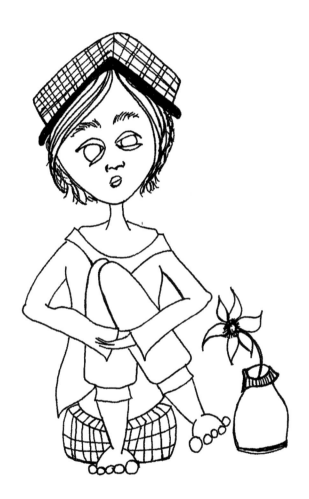

Om or Aum (ॐ) is a sound without beginning or end.
The sound pulsing through the universe.
The sound of the divine and peace and stillness.
Sing...
Tune your wisdom eye and the vibrations of your heart.

Sound the Quiet

Om is a sacred sound, a *mantra*, widely used in meditation practices. It is said that ancient sages heard the sound of Om when their thoughts were quiet and still. Can you hear the hum of Om as an airplane flies overhead, on a windy day, when it rains, when the stars shine? With practice you can hear Om beneath your thoughts, words, and actions.

Meditation

Sit comfortably, lengthen your spine, and lift your heart. Your chin is parallel to the ground. You might soften your gaze, looking at nothing solid. And if you feel safe, you might close your eyes all the way. Let them relax behind relaxed lids. Feel strong but relaxed.

Begin *Three-Part Breathing* to create the physical space for your breath to slow down. Here you are starting to tune your mind, like the volume of your music, adjusting the noises outside of you, lower, if possible, so you can drop into stillness.

Inhale deep (fill your belly, ribs, and chest); as you exhale, give voice to the sound of "AHHH," opening your mouth wide, then make an O with your lips saying "UUUU," close your lips as you hum "MMMM."

Chant Om (AHHH, UUUU, MMMM) each time you exhale. Try to feel the quiet when you inhale. Let there be no separation between your chanting the vibrations of Om in your throat and breathing. Imagine that you are riding with the sound on your bike, in an airplane, on your skateboard; you are the sound moving through light and time.

Do this for nine rounds, and then just listen and feel the movement of the tone through you. With practice, you might hear the vibrations of your voice in this quiet space. Your voice has the support of the universe; let's keep tapping into this infinite resource, fine-tuning your gifts.

Attune to Center

For you to be able to come into the space of your center, everything else has to drop away. Your center is: who you are, not what you do, or who you might become, but it is you now.

You will need a candle for this centering meditation.

Meditation

Sit comfortably with a long spine, relax your shoulders, and lift your heart. Light a candle, place it about two or three feet in front of you. Sit the flame lower than your eye level so you can gaze upon it with half-closed, or half-opened, eyes.

Close your eyes, and do three rounds of *Alternate Nostril Breathing*— this technique balances your sides, getting you closer to your center. Begin by pulling air into your LEFT nostril and end your third, last round of this breathwork by exhaling out of your LEFT nostril.

Open your eyelids halfway; immediately focus on the candle flame. Breathe smoothly and deeply. Keep looking at the flame. Focus on the flame. You may blink a lot. Be patient. Your eyes may burn. Keep focusing. You might produce tears, cleaning your eyes. Focus. The flame might get bigger, smaller, wave back and forth, wiggle. Watch through your mind's eye; draw the flame in the center of the candle into your center.

Soften your focus even more, and feel the flame filling your heart with light as it warms you. Close your eyes all the way, and feel as if you have become the flame, and the flame is you burning strongly and shining brightly. As the image of the flame begins to fade, gently blink your eyes open.

Sit still for a few rounds of breath. Feel steady on the surface beneath you. Move slowly away from this space, holding you.

Move to Stillness

Dancing as meditation can help you express who you are and what you are feeling in a given moment. You will need music for this practice and enough room to spread your wings.

Meditation

Stand tall in *Mountain* pose. Begin *Ocean Breathing*, swelling and deflating your belly with each breath. Listen to the movement of your breath. Can you see it in your mind's eye? Can you feel its rhythm?

Imagine the journey the air you're taking in is making as it cycles through your body. Let's move with this freedom and find your unique waltz.

You might count (three on one side, three in the opposite direction) when you begin your circles, but eventually release the counts and feel into your natural movements. Circle your head (be gentle with your neck) in one direction, then the other. Roll your shoulders front, up, back, down, then back, up, front, down, to begin the process of loosening all you might be holding. Open and close your fingers; invite your wrists to the party—circle them in, out, up, down. Snake your arms from side to side, moving through your shoulders as a belly dancer might. Circle your hips in one direction, then the other. Bring your movements together slowly as if you are meeting a new friend, then grow bigger and freer.

Feel your breath and feel the music. Listen with your entire body. Make your breath match the music (fast or slow, high or low). Try to express what you feel. Move your dance from your center. Feel your movements coming from your center space.

Dance from the inside, out. Bring your outside dance inward, especially if you have felt sad or heavy for a period of time. Life is a constant dance of balance; don't get stuck, be flexible at times, rooted in others. You are a part of the universe's rhythm (remember Om). Learning to harmonize your flow with our shared community is an important part of the work of yoga.

As your dance begins to slow and you feel stillness stronger than the music or your movements, close your eyes. Turn your palms up toward the sky with a soft bend in your elbows. Lift your heart and gaze upward. Embrace the freedom of expressing who you are at your center.

CHAPTER 12

Making Stuff that Matters

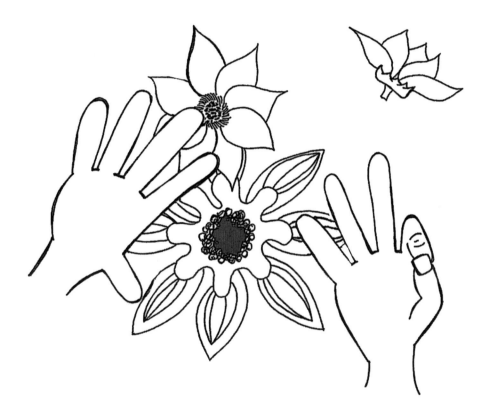

Create your world, breath by breath,
moment to moment, and project by project.
Practice. Revise. Practice again. Live.

My Cosmic Pond

Close your eyes and bring your awareness to your wisdom eye. How do you envision your cosmic pond: the result of your thoughts, words, and actions, and other stuff beyond your control?

Supplies

* heavy paper

* environmentally kind wall adhesive (*you may want to change the background eventually, or move to a new space*)

* imagination

Project

To explore your cosmic pond, get a large length of art paper or several poster sheets that will cover your wall. Allow room for the world you are designing to grow and expand.

Your drawings can be complex, layered with shading and cross-hatching, or peopled with stick figures and primitive representations; this is your (secret, natural) code. Add to it each time you receive something new from your gut or from the world outside you: something important whether it seems large or extremely small.

Draw (in words and pictures) the world you see.

Examine what affects you from the outside (stuff you didn't invite, persistent stuff that doesn't feel comfortable or right at first) by carrying it around (like you carry the things in your book bag or purse) with your thoughts (your innerness) for a few hours or days. Upon waking, say "Good morning" to you. Notice how you feel: *mostly good, OK, or very good*.

Then present the stuff you've been gnawing on, one at a time; decide how you feel, first response, make a mental note. Let go of these gems, sinkholes, and mountains, and move into your day.

See, feel, and decide what this stuff, especially if it's new, really means to you before adding it to your wall art. *Is it stuff you really need? Are these circumstances you want to manifest—to come true?*

Keep looking at the persistent stuff, the *it bugs me* stuff that just doesn't fit into any category, through your wisdom eye. Go to your wall. *Can you see it in your pond? How is it settling within your world and your imaginings? Does your stomach feel upset as you consider the ripples it might make? Are you excited about including it in your day?*

Keep asking: *How does this serve me and the people, places, and things around me?*

If you decide the new stuff serves you, add it to your wall in pencil at first; live with this new view a while longer. Ask again: *Does it fit me? My worldview?*

If your head and heart convince you that it does not fit (*it just doesn't feel good*), erase it to make room for what feels more like you. Notice when your cosmic pond is agitated, notice when it's calm.

What I See Today

Hold this view intentionally for a few moments each day.

Zine Designing

A zine is a small-circulation publication of original, remixed, and remade content. Create your own zine from front to back, shaping the content in between, then photocopy, scan, or email it to your friends and selected audience. Leave it where other people can pick it up: the cafeteria, the girls' room, your website, your favorite coffee shop, at the farmer's market, near the entrance of the public library. Make it about what you want to share and think the masses need to know. What have you learned about the world, your school, your neighborhood? About you (though this is not your diary or *cosmic pond* wall—places for your deepest secrets) and how you relate to your environs? What are your specialties and gifts? How can you translate them into pictures and words and present them in a way that others will read, remember, and pass on? Cover what you would change about the world, but don't turn your zine into a whining baby others will get tired of reading because it does not offer dreams.

Design, make, and share your zine.

Supplies

* how-to-do (do-it-yourself) tips for things you've mastered

* commentary on why a book you read is interesting

* imagination, interesting images, prose and poetry that stick with you (remember to include the name of the author if you use someone else's work)

* photocopier or scanner or computer access

Project

Name your zine (something important to you or others in your community), determine your subject, and start producing a publication that might help people understand each other better.

Your zine content should include your writing, drawing, and creativity.

Cover the front and back of a single piece of paper with your content, make copies (with a scanner or photocopier, or by hand), and distribute.

Zine Canvas

_____

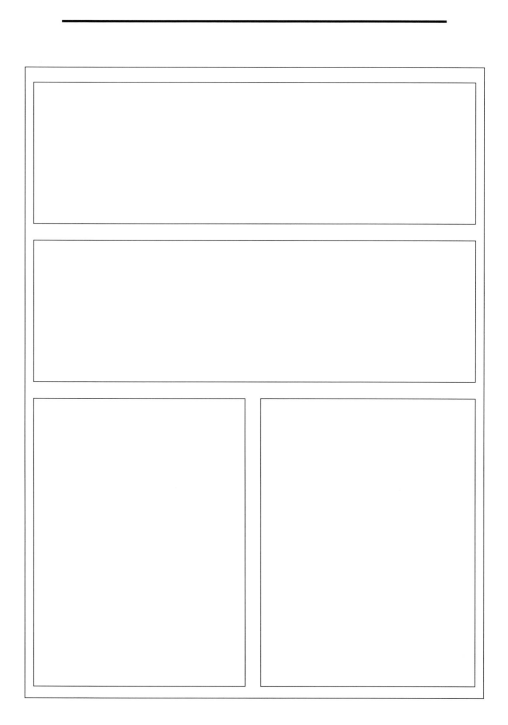

Yogini Making

When you were younger, did you ever play with dolls that you made or cut out of paper? Did they talk to each other or, better yet, to you? Did you make only one of a kind, like designers make some styles, unique like you? Did you place them in strange scenarios and situations? Whether you did or did not, now is the time to make a *yogini* (a girl similar to you, who does yoga) with movable parts, so she can practice her yoga postures. You can design a cool wardrobe and accessories for this amazing girl. Add on whatever you think she might need as she moves through your days with you.

Supplies

* heavy paper (card stock); sturdy decorative paper with patterns and colors that speak to you; lightweight paper; graphic-rich fabrics; ribbon; any material you can bend or give shape to create your *yogini*

* scissors

* writing/drawing utensils

* brads (silver, gold)—a top with two prongs or legs that separate (they are often used to fasten paper together)

Project

Draw and cut out your *yogini* parts: head with attached torso, two upper arms with attached shoulder and elbow, two lower arms with attached elbow and hand, two upper legs with attached knee cap, two lower legs with attached knee and foot. As you design your girl, use the *yogini* pattern as inspiration (it's on p.160). Push brads through the overlapping body parts: head to neck, upper arm to torso, lower arm to upper arm, thigh to torso, and lower leg to thigh.

As you work make sure your *yogini* is fabulous; model her on your best qualities, especially those you don't always believe you possess.

Variation

Once you've mastered making a paper *yogini*, explore changing your medium (the main material or form used by an artist). You might make a fabric *yogini*—basically, the limbs will be the same, but you will assemble them from your favorite textiles.

Fabric Yogini

Cut out:

two heads	four lower arms
two torsos	four thighs
four upper arms	four lower legs

Sew front to back, and part to part (head to neck, upper arm to torso, lower arm to upper arm, thigh to torso, and lower leg to thigh), stuffing her with cotton, rice, or beads.

You could even make a *yogini* out of polymer clay. Shape and sculpt your *yogini*. Put in some recessed places near her joints especially, so she can be flexible when she feels hard knocks or bumps in her days. Use toothpicks to make holes in her connecting parts (head, neck and torso, shoulder, elbow, hip, and knee joints) and then string them together with something strong such as fishing line.

Over time, can you see your attempts to live yogic-ly (practicing your poses regularly, working on breathing techniques, making time to meditate, living from the kind space inside you, even as you work to balance in the face of conflict and challenge) reflecting in her?

Yogini Pattern

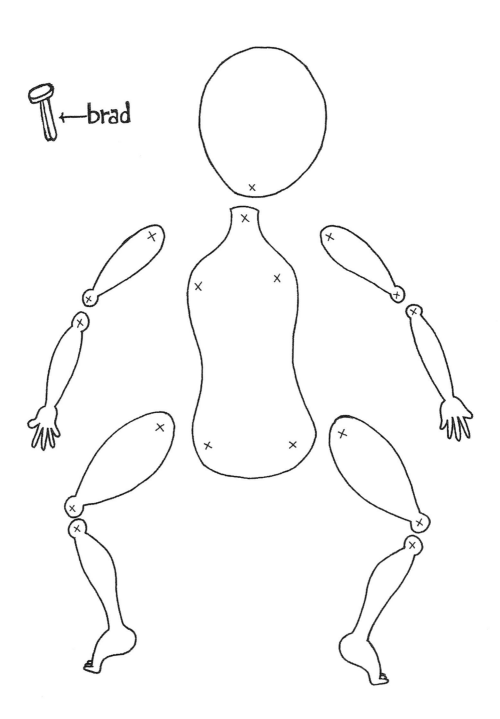

Clothes for your Yogini

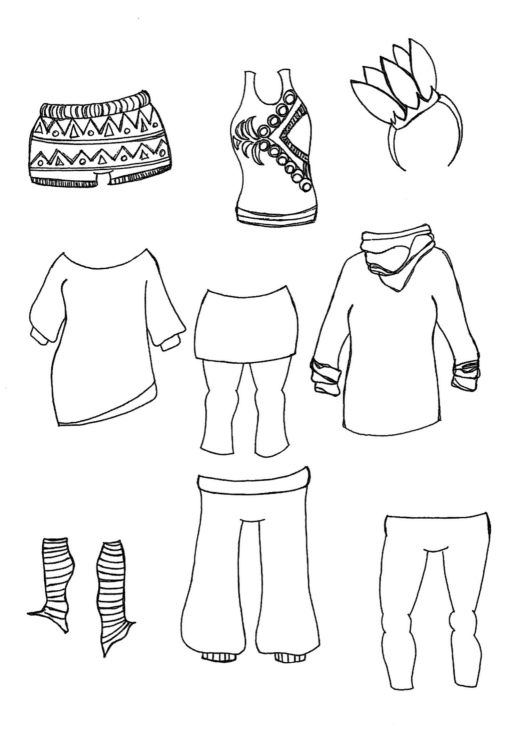

Mala Making

A mala is a string of beads, made with 108, 54, or 27 beads, useful in meditation, when concentrating, or for wearing as a reminder of the goodness at your center. Twenty-seven (2+7=9), 54 (5+4=9), and 108 (1+0+8=9) all equal nine, a perfect number in yoga, which invites success. Nine is associated with the range of emotions, moods, and modes of creative expression. Nine is also linked to the number of human desires and planets that rule astrological signs and outcomes.

When you make a mala, add an extra bead that is different from the others, symbolizing the teacher within. This is the *guru bead*, representing that you are your own best guide when you open to what there is to learn in your experiences.

Use your mala to mark the rhythm of your breath or to guide your repetition of your *mantra*. Use it to remind you of you at any given moment (when you encounter conflict, or experience extreme happiness, as well as in all of the daily spaces between these opposites).

Necklace Supplies

* stiff thread or sturdy string

* 108 beads

* one *guru bead*

* one tassel (optional)

Bracelet Supplies

* stretchy cord

* 27 beads

* one *guru bead*

* one tassel (optional)

Project

For a necklace, hold the end of the cord in one hand and unwind it with your other hand; so with your arms opened wide, make sure it extends from one of your hands to the other. For a bracelet, use stretchy cord half as long.

If you are using a tassel, thread your cord through the tassel leaving yourself a tail about two inches long. You will hide your knot here when you are finished stringing your beads. Without the tassel, secure the end in a loose knot, or under a strong piece of tape fastened to a flat surface (so the beads do not fall off as you string them).

Next, put your *guru bead* on your cord and string the rest of your beads (108 for a necklace, 27 for a bracelet).

Once all your beads are strung, tie the free end to the inch-long tail.

Make a few knots, securing one on top of the other, so your knot will not come undone. Hide your knot within the tassel.

Note: if you are making a bracelet with stretchy cord, do not pull so hard that you remove the stretch out of it. Tie it so your beads fit snugly, and the bracelet stretches when you put it on your wrist.

Cut any extra cord to an inch and tuck it into your guru bead and two or three beads next to it, and snip the ends. Or let them hang long and cut them to the same length as your tassel.

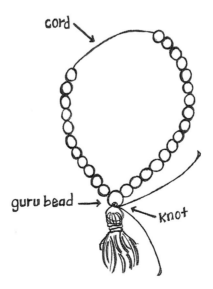

Defeating Your Gremlin(s)

When negative and nasty thoughts start to creep into your mental space, it is probably not "good you," but your gremlin acting out; everyone has one. Search your imagination: can you see your evil insider? If you can see, or hear, or smell it, give it a name that describes its most flaming traits. It only has power if you give it power, and it is probably upset because you have been ignoring it.

Sometimes your gremlin will overpower you with its contributions, but you are not your gremlin, and your gremlin is not all of you. It is just a voice complaining, a negative force trying to keep you from being your best self and living your dreams.

If you can keep this in mind, your gremlin becomes just another something that might show up when you are feeling unsure or trying something new. Nevertheless, you are stronger than it, even if it visits you often. It has no real power; recognize its presence, and let it make its complaints quietly, then tell it to go away. So you can move beyond its control.

Supplies

* paper

* drawing pencils

* colored pencils or markers

Project

Bring your gremlin to life. Give it a solid form. Draw it.

Now it's outside of you, no longer a part of you (for now); you have won this battle.

Notice when your gremlin appears and what it does when it shows up. How does its appearances affect how you feel, and affect what you do? Does it stand in front of your possibilities like a roadblock, or stop sign, or towering mountain? What can you do to overcome your gremlin and people who act like your gremlin by trying to make you feel bad about yourself or never quite good enough?

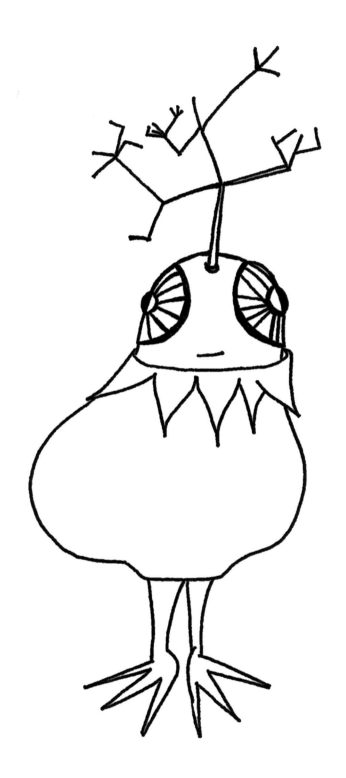

You Can Draw Your Gremlin
It Can't Draw You

Recognize when your gremlin is on the attack.
You are the strongest. You are stronger than it.

Mask Making

A mask is a covering that can both hide your identity and show people different sides of you. A mask can personify aspects of yourself that you choose to show to the world; a mask can hide parts of you that you decide are just for you. This can be a tricky balancing act.

Like yoga, using one mask and seeing behind the masks of others is an intentional practice. Make your mask often, daily, weekly. We change every minute, hour, day. Who do you most want to be?

Supplies

* drawing pencils

* colored pencils and markers

* sparkles, paint, fabric, glue

Project

When you close your eyes, how do you see your face? Hold the image in your mind's eye and create a mask that reflects what you see, how you see it. Think of this mask as showing *you* in this moment. The *you* only you can see.

Hold the mask you created beside your face as you look at your reflection in a mirror. How does the face you see in the mirror compare with the mask you made? Use seven or more descriptive words, a combination of physical traits and emotions you might be feeling, and experiencing.

How do you think other people see you? List some words that others might use to describe you:

_____, _____, _____, _____,

_____, _____, and _____.

Do you agree with these? Are they an accurate reflection of you?

Using this list, make another mask; this one is from an outsider's point of view. *How would this girl look? The one others see when they look at me today?*

How are your masks similar, how are they different? Which mask shows a truer reflection of you right now?

How I See Myself

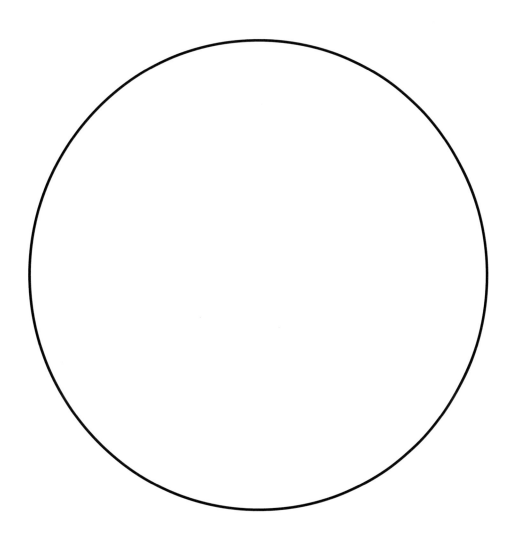

How I Think Others See Me

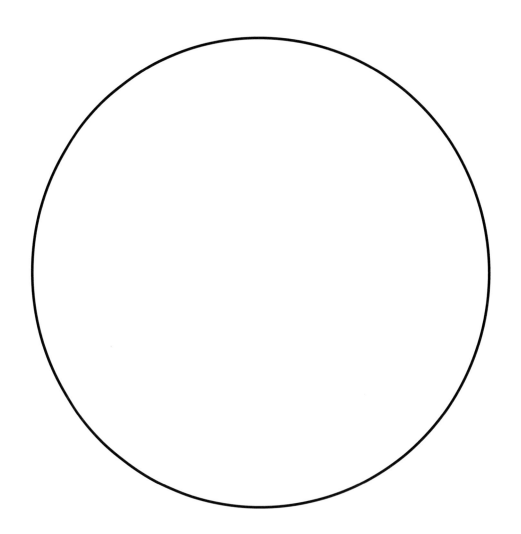

Haiku Writing

Originating in Japanese writing, a haiku is a form of poetry consisting of three lines and 17 syllables. Often inspired by nature and your experiences, haikus are capable of creating images to help you see your ideas in words.

The first line of three consists of five syllables, the second line is seven syllables, and the third line is five syllables.

Supplies

* pencil or pen

* a journal to collect your writings, so you can begin to notice if there are recurring patterns

Project

Write a story about yourself in a series of haikus, connecting each haiku to the one before it by repeating a word, sound, or idea. Choose an important event in your life and focus on the three important parts that made the experience meaningful.

Focus on three parts of your community, such as your route to school, aspects or oddities of your favorite sport, or of your favorite food. Weave in the things that stand out about these subjects. Your haikus should show you some interesting connections about yourself and your community.

1st Haiku

_____

_____

_____

2nd Haiku

_____

_____

_____

3rd Haiku

_____

_____

_____

Dreamscapes

To make your dreams come true, you have to believe in them, breathe life into them by faithfully spending time every day, visualizing them happening. Think about the things and realities that are most important to you; what are they? See them in your mind's eye; try to focus on the overall vision rather than the details, because the particulars are often different in the actualization of a dream, while the essence of the dream remains in its truest form when it walks into the sunlight or starshine of your life.

You can make your dreams come true by connecting your goals and actions with your *dharma*. Each day brings the opportunity to get to know yourself better, to discover your gifts, and how you are supposed to share them with the world—which feeds your own growth.

If you can imagine something, water and fertilize and love it as you would your favorite plants; it will grow and bloom when the time is right and your moment meets your preparation (tending your dream garden) and luck in a way that feels perfectly right.

If you can recognize your own potential and stay alert to all that is possible and finding its way to you from the universe of your good, you will begin to move toward it, effecting and living into your dreams. You are one of the greatest guardians of your dreams.

Supplies

* paper

* drawing pencils

* colored pencils and markers

Project

Make your dreams a reality through your intentional use of action words (usually verbs) and images (usually something that affects your five senses and begins to travel with you, something meaningful to you, that you can't explain or see fully yet, but that feels important) to make your dreams real.

Draw, write, doodle, color—capture your dream bit by bit—make some magic.

Real to Real

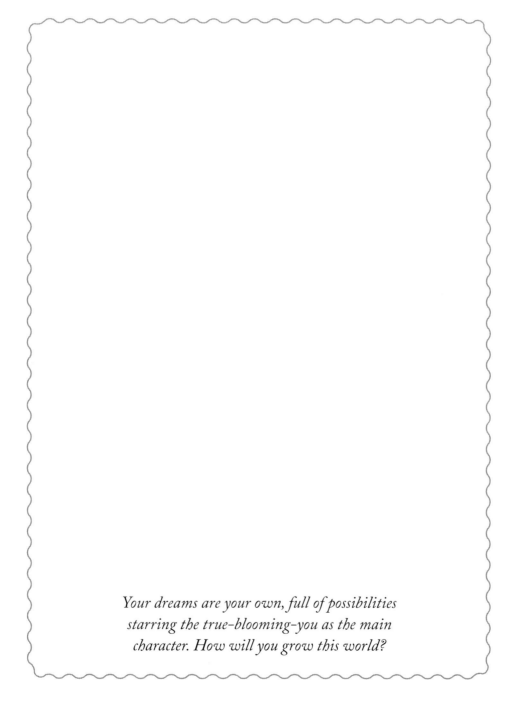

*Your dreams are your own, full of possibilities
starring the true-blooming-you as the main
character. How will you grow this world?*

CHAPTER 13

Yogini Being

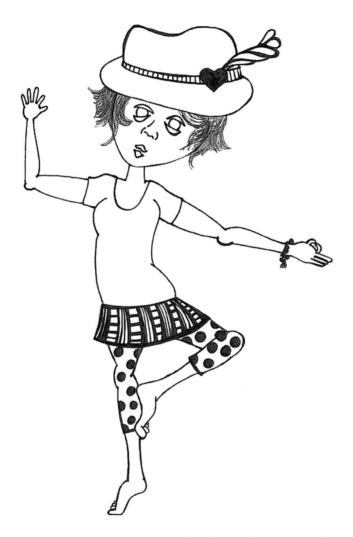

Your yoga practice transcends the walls you or others
create, connecting your thoughts, words, and actions
to your movements and the way you live on earth.

What is a Yogini?

Practicing yoga encompasses breathing fully, speaking your truth calmly with an awareness of what you believe is true, and living and acting in ways that contribute to our collective well-being (when life can be as right as it can be for as many as it can be). Yoga extends beyond postures, breathing with awareness, and meditating. The practice of yoga is about how you see and interact with the world. Practicing yoga is continuous, difficult at times, daily, joy-filled work.

When you live your yoga, you are in the space of being yourself from the inside out. In your zone, your perceptions of the world and your place in it become expansive, making room for you to think inspired, creative thoughts, and dream limitless possibilities as you live your days. As you wake to the new morning, say: *I'm here, present*, and "become" whatever you deserve and expect and dream of "being."

When you are aware that you can transcend (leap over or through) all boundaries, you can be yourself from your inmost place of peace (though you might have to yogic-ly outwait some circumstances). A girl who embodies as many parts of her yoga practice as possible is a *yogini*. As a *yogini*, you recognize the brightness of your light, even in your darkest moments. No matter what, you will not give this light away to fit into circles where you cannot see your good, to take the easier path that everyone around you seems to be traveling, or to get something quickly that you do not really need to possess.

Recognizing that: when light meets light, it merges with the other light to become even brighter, and even when light meets darkness or is cast with shadows, light shines just as brightly, a *yogini* shines the light of who she is in all she does, makes, and works toward becoming.

You are a *yogini*, a yoga girl, a creative, expressive being, an integral part of this world. Try to be your best you in everything you do. Accept yourself. Be OK with your reality, as you believe in all of your possibilities.

Yogini State of Mind

You've been practicing yoga regularly in your own space; now it's time to explore how your personal practice moves and breathes and feels out in the world.

Outside your own space, you have to zoom in on your inner compass, commit to everything you have discovered about the way your body moves into the postures, feel confident in the way your mind knows and can sense what feels right in your muscles, bones, and joints. With this awareness, be flexible and open to what is out there, similar to the fluidity of your *Warrior II* when you can bend deeper into your front knee, making your thigh more parallel to the ground. But in this openness to learning more, you're not going to give away the truth of what you've learned about you. This is the supreme balancing act: *how do I stay true to myself in interaction with others?*

There are many different types of yoga, but you possess a strong foundation that you can use to explore the yoga practices that work for you and rule out those that do not, whether you are in a class at school, a studio, the gym, or anywhere else. Avoid experiences that do not feel right because it is too easy to hurt yourself by practicing in the wrong ways. You know how to stack your joints, starfish your fingers to support your *Downward-Facing Dog*, how to align your neck with your spine as you look slightly forward at the earth in *Four-Limbed Staff*. If you cannot avoid settings that do not feel right, "*practice your own practice*" with respect: if the instructor cues *Balancing Half Moon*, do it at the same time, but use what you've worked on to build a safe pose. *Do you need a block under your bottom hand to lift the floor up to meet you? Do you need to keep your top hand on your hip to feel more stable? What do you need to do to make this pose and the others fit you?*

Do not lose your yoga practice in this new environment.

Practicing in a public setting can be rewarding and tricky. If you have questions, ask them when the right time presents itself. If you find a place to practice regularly, you should feel comfortable with the setting (like in your *Downward-Facing Dog*) and at ease with the people practicing with you.

Most importantly, listen to you. *You know yourself best. You are your own best guide.*

Yogini Manifesto

The definition of "manifest": to display or show (a quality or feeling) by one's acts or appearance. See your hands moving your thoughts and intentions in positive ways to show, to achieve your dreams, and to impact your community.

A manifesto is a declaration of who you know you are and of the things that are important to you. It is your philosophy. These words are personal. They inspire you to be yourself, to keep growing your garden, as you co-create our world.

Write your manifesto in affirmative, positive, and kind language using the present tense.

Record your responses to these questions:

* What do you think about you, right now?

* What's on your cosmic pond wall? Does it agree?

* Do most of your actions match what you believe?

* Do you direct your mind toward your actions and beliefs regularly?

* Do you have goals for your future? What are they?

* Do you visualize them every day, or every few days?

This is an evolving conversation.

Project

Use your answers to create your philosophy.

Use the *My Manifesto* structure to make your declarations and chart your own course, so you can sail in the directions that are best for you.

Read your manifesto often; add to it, and revise your statements as you come to know more and more about yourself and what you believe and continue to hold as important as you live your days.

Your manifesto will change and evolve as you do, but there will be aspects of it that always remain the same. You might find that these say the most about you, and form the unchanging constants of your truth. These are the parts of you that fill you with your unique light.

My Manifesto

I am _____

_____

_____

I do _____

_____

_____

I make _____

_____

_____

I am becoming _____

_____

_____

Your manifesto is alive. It grows and changes with you.
Revisit and revise it as often as you need so it always reflects you.

Taking Yoga Classes

When you participate in yoga experiences out in the community, you have to carry the knowledge of what you have come to know about yourself and your practice of yoga with you like a piece of jewelry you'd never leave home without. This knowledge encompasses what you know to be true—who you are, what you need, and how you practice. Above all else, you are your own best guide.

Do what you can do, how you can do it, no matter what the person next to you, in front of you, or behind you might be doing. Listen to your body and your intuition as you open yourself up to experiencing what is being presented.

If something does not feel right in the environment, in your body, in your mind—don't do it.

This might mean modifying a posture your own way, quietly sitting on your mat and not doing something being instructed if you are not comfortable with it (not because it is difficult or new to you or because you don't think you can, but because you are giving yourself the latitude not to do something if it does not feel right in your gut, in your soul, from your point of view). Maybe even in some cases you will respectfully remove yourself from the situation.

Your body and mind have their own language: look, listen, feel into what they're saying and experiencing.

Your practice of yoga should be something you enjoy. Pick and choose the classes you take in accordance with what makes you feel good while inspiring you to be your best self.

Likewise, don't "short change" yourself: you should feel good as you push your boundaries, expanding your limbs and petals through your world.

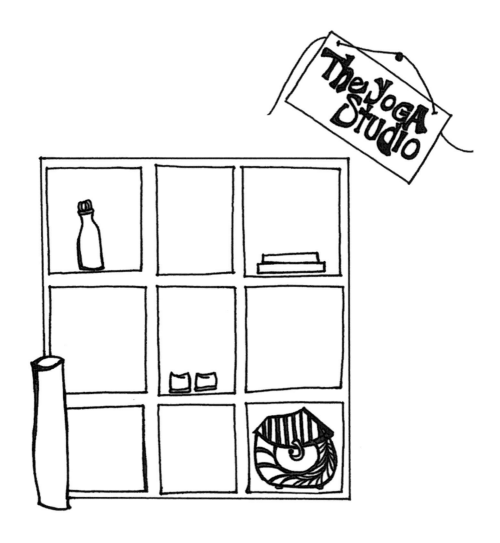

Yoga Class Checklist

Before you go, know:

- ✳ When, where, and how long the class will last.

- ✳ What type of class you are taking.

- ✳ How much the class costs.

Take with you:

 ✳ Payment to cover the cost of the class.

 ✳ A yoga mat (or be prepared to borrow or rent one, possibly for a fee).

 ✳ Layers of clothing, in case you get cold or hot, and water to drink.

Getting there:

 ✳ Arrive at least ten minutes early to get a feel for the space and complete any necessary paperwork (usually waivers related to your physical health). Fifteen minutes early is ideal.

When you're there:

 ✳ Use your five senses to investigate the place; does the energy of the space give you good vibes?

 ✳ If there are shoes and socks by the door, in cubby holes, or against the back wall of the room, leave yours there too.

 ✳ If the environment feels safe, place your personal items off to the side; otherwise place your stuff behind or near your yoga mat.

 ✳ Silence your electronic devices; ideally leave them outside your practice space.

 ✳ Focus past distractions and remember the *you* you brought to class and the journey *you're* on.

Types of Yoga

A lot of the time we like to categorize and name things so we can understand them and figure out how we will interact with them. While the types of yoga are relevant, they don't really matter as much as incorporating the practices that make you feel good about yourself into your daily life.

The names and the teachers of yoga vary, but yoga is yoga. Explore the variations and settle into a practice that challenges you, inspires you, and holds your attention.

The Petals You Will Bring to Every Practice

You are your own best guide; you are your guru; *listen to the messages and the feelings that come from deep inside you when practicing yoga. Listen to yourself. Be respectful of the environment; even if you have to leave, do it as peacefully as possible. Different people are at different points on our shared path.*

The different types of yoga focus on varying aspects of the practice. The yoga of postures and breath is *Hatha*, balancing the hot fast energy of the sun (ha) with the cool calm energy of the moon (tha).

Jnana is the yoga of universal knowledge, revolving around the connection between yourself and everything.

Bhakti is the yoga of love and service to God.

Karma yoga is the path of action where you serve others.

Raja is the yoga of controlling your mind and emotions through meditation and contemplation.

Don't worry about deciding what kind of *yogini* you are or picking just one type of yoga to practice because all the forms of yoga are connected. You will feel this as you bloom in your practice. Throughout history, great sages and saints have said, "The paths are many, the truth is one."

Styles of Yoga

These are the most widely practiced styles of yoga you might find in various interpretations in your local community.

* *Ashtanga Yoga*—a series of postures incorporating jumping forward and back with *vinyasa* flows between postures. This type of yoga is based on opposites, designed to fold your spine forward and bend your spine back. A traditional *Ashtanga* class does not usually include music. During a practice you might feel your muscles contracting and stretching, talking to you loudly; afterwards you may notice or feel the sensation of longness, new length in your body. Or you might feel sore in certain joints, limbs, and muscles.

* *Hot Yoga*—a sequenced series of postures practiced in a heated room. This heat can be like hot oil with temperatures upwards of 90 degrees. The heat makes you feel extra stretchy and bendy because it warms your muscles from the outside, rather than you easing into their depth with stretches that warm you from the inside so you can expand out. Generally you will know if you are stretching too far by the way your body feels during the practice, and the next day. Yes, you want to challenge yourself, working into the abilities of your body, maybe feeling things you've never felt before, but when you feel pain—shooting, ripping, ouch-inducing trauma—stop what you are doing and find a way to do the pose without pain.

* *Vinyasa* or *Flow Yoga*—movements synchronized to your inhalation and exhalation: your breath. Generally, one posture will transition into the next. Most likely this style will appeal to you if you like to dance (or wish you could dance) because the movement of your body is constant and rhythmic. Music plays a major role in these classes as well. After you practice *Vinyasa* or *Flow* style for a while, see if the music can help you connect your movements and your mind space.

✳ *Kundalini Yoga*—focuses on the movement of your energy through the major energy centers, your *chakras*, which dot the spine from your tailbone to the crown of your head. To move your energy, *Kundalini* yoga typically involves chanting and repetitive movements called *kriyas*. Channeling the energy through your *chakras* can help you relieve stress, relax your mind, and improve your memory. The claim: if you are able to uncoil the energy at the base of your spine and move it up from your most primal desires (eating, sleeping, thinking about sex), you can tap into your higher realms of consciousness and achieve bliss.

✳ *Yin Yoga*—involves remaining in a posture for a while (anywhere from three to ten minutes is normal). The idea is: if you are in a posture for a long time without worrying about holding your body a certain way, gravity will slowly work you deeper into the pose, targeting a stretch in the deep muscles of the body. As you fold over the diamond shape of your legs in *Butterfly*, you might begin by using a yoga block on its highest height to support your head. After two minutes or so, as you feel more space in your inner thighs and more length in your spine, you might place the block on a lower height, allowing your head to drop closer to your feet. Afterwards, you may experience different sensations, soreness, and stronger and heightened alertness in your muscles and a quieter, more reflective state of mind.

There are many styles of yoga, ancient and newly emerging; whatever forms you end up exploring, always check in with yourself and ask: *Does this agree with my physical and mental body? Listen to your inner voice, your answers.*

Namaste

Namaste is the Sanskrit word and gesture of greeting and parting. In yoga it means: "The spirit and light in me honors and acknowledges the spirit and light in you."

Press your palms together in front of your heart. Gently press your thumbs to the center of your chest. Imagine your heart rising up beyond your palms.

Bow your head toward your heart, closing your eyes to everything outside you, opening them wide to the light within you. See the light in your heart; you are the only one who can shine it into the world.

In your mind's eye, acknowledge the light of others; we are all so different, yet connected, and in many ways the same.

Honor and acknowledge the light within you. Like the most exquisite diamond, with bold cuts and artistry that attracts earthshine and reflects the beauty they share, you have many, many facets. Yoga can help you with the work and fun of getting to know yourself. Illumine the world, with your light. Keep fueling your light with energy. Shine in all you say, do, create, and become.

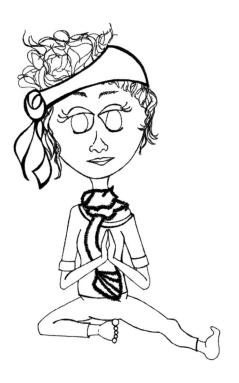

GLOSSARY

Asanas: yoga postures or positions. You'll notice that most of the posture names end with "asana," like: *Tadasana* (*Mountain Pose*), *Sukhasana* (*Comfortable Seat*), and *Savasana* (*Relaxation Pose*).

Chakras: spinning centers of energy throughout the body, there are seven main ones located along the centerline of your body, from your tailbone to your crown.

Consciousness: being awake and aware of who you are.

Cosmic pond: the collection of your thoughts, words, and actions (and all the other stuff too).

Cosmos: the universe, all existing matter and space considered as a whole.

Cultivate: grow something as a part of you; grow "*you*" as a part of the universe.

Dharma: identifying the best way for you to live your life.

Devotion: deeply seated love, loyalty, and belief in something.

Dristhi: where you focus your eye gaze; a steady focus can often improve your balance and sense of stability.

Embrace: accept and believe in something entirely; this generally precedes *devotion*.

Faith: holding the belief that the things, concepts, and dreams you hope will come true will become real; believing in what you cannot see (yet).

Ground: connecting to the earth with whatever part (feet, hands, seat) of you that is meeting it in your pose.

Guru: an influential teacher or spiritual guide; the letters make the phrase "g-you-are-you." You will have many teachers, some excellent, some bad, but remember your feelings and intuition are often your best guides.

Haiku: a form of poetry consisting of 17 syllables written in three lines; the first line consists of five syllables, the second line seven syllables, and the third line five syllables.

Intention: focuses on the present moment, a positive thought you use to guide your efforts.

Karma: how your thoughts, words, and actions influence your life; how intentions influence your present and your future.

Mala: a string of beads used for meditation, concentration, and recitation of a mantra or prayer.

Mantra: a sound, word, or a phrase that when repeated frequently can help you become calm; it can help focus your thinking in preparation for meditation. If your thoughts are scattered, a mantra can help you let anything you need float by like clouds in the sky, so you can become clear.

Mudras: gestures that can influence your energy and mood; most often made with your hands and fingers, although they can involve any part or all of the body.

Om: the sound of stillness, of the quiet under, over, around, and in all things. It is the humming vibration of the universe connecting everything and all of us.

Prana: your energy and life force, present in each and every breath you take.

Sanskrit: an ancient language spoken in India around 1200–1400 BC.

Shakti: the feminine divine energy inside all of us; your creative power.

Shiva: the masculine divine energy inside all of us; this is your power to make things, but also to destroy them in order to rebuild them again.

Stuff that matters: the things that make you smile from the inside out, as you shine bright with happy, hopeful, creative energy; what you feel passionate about without knowing why you feel so intensely about it.

Surrender: letting go of how or what you think should be right now, and opening up a space for what is in the present.

Third eye: the home of your intuition, things that you know but you do not always know why you know them, or how you know them. The third eye houses your sixth sense.

Vinyasa: placing your body in a special way, guided by your inhalation and exhalation; also a series of postures linked together in movements that flow from one to the next as you take breath in and release it.

Wisdom: learning from your experiences.

Yogini: a girl who practices yoga in her thoughts, words, and actions.